Fundamentals of
Regional
Anaesthesia

Fundamentals of
Regional
Anaesthesia

H.B.J. Fischer
C.A. Pinnock

Department of Anaesthesia
Alexandra Hospital
Woodrow Drive
Redditch
Worcestershire
UK

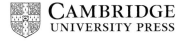
CAMBRIDGE
UNIVERSITY PRESS

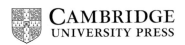

© 2004

Cambridge University Press

ISBN 1 841 10126 5

First Published 2004

A catalogue record for this book is available from the British Library.

Project Manager: Gavin Smith

Typeset by Charon Tec Pvt. Ltd, Chennai, India
www.charontec.com
Printed in the UK by Cambridge University Press

Preface

This book was written primarily for trainee anaesthetists with an interest in regional anaesthesia but it may also benefit more experienced medical staff who would like to learn new techniques or update their skills. Over the last 20 years, at the Alexandra Hospital in Redditch, we have taught several generations of trainee anaesthetists in the practical skills of peripheral and central neural blockade. In fact, it is due to the suggestions of many of those trainees that we have committed ourselves to publishing our approach to regional anaesthesia. This book is a distillation of our teaching and practice of regional anaesthesia, and is designed to complement supervision by an experienced mentor, rather than act as a 'do it yourself' manual. Inexperienced practitioners should seek expert advice when performing a nerve block for the first time, especially if the technique is complex.

We strongly advise newcomers to the field of regional anaesthesia to study the contents of Section 1, 'Principles and practice' before performing any of the nerve blocks described later in the book. This section outlines the benefits of regional anaesthesia and our philosophy of how best to incorporate these benefits into your practice. Details on the contraindications and complications of regional anaesthesia, safety aspects and the precautions for safeguarding patient welfare are summarised. A brief description of the pharmacology of local anaesthetic drugs is also included and we make no apologies for stressing the need for resuscitation skills and equipment, and intravenous access (even in minor procedures).

Section 2, 'Peripheral nerve blocks', is arranged in a logical manner from the lower limb through the abdomen, the thorax and the upper limb to the head and neck. It provides a comprehensive overview of the applied anatomy of the peripheral somatic nerve supply of the body and guidance as to which peripheral nerve blocks are suitable for the intended surgical procedure. This allows the reader to revise the nerve supply to a particular operative site and select suitable nerve blocks in advance of a surgical list. This section describes in detail a full range of peripheral nerve blocks for all major areas of the body. For consistency, the right-sided approach is always used.

Section 3, 'Central neuraxial blocks', describes the central neuraxial anatomy, surgical indications and major central nerve blocks in a similar layout to Section 2. Line and perspective diagrams to clarify and define the skills required for each technique complement the written descriptions. This is in line with our philosophy that successful regional anaesthesia depends on identifying the key topographical landmarks and refining the necessary needle movements to a minimum. By distilling out the essential core of information for each nerve block technique, the likelihood of early success with a new technique is enhanced and the risks of morbidity and complication can be minimised.

The drugs and volumes of solution listed with each technique are for general guidance only (based on a standard 70 kg patient). The actual concentration and volume of a drug administered to an individual patient must be based on their specific needs. Maximum dose guidelines for each local anaesthetic should not be exceeded and if combinations of local anaesthetics are used, the maximum doses are cumulative not additive. Bupivacaine is used to illustrate the maximum duration of effect but shorter-acting agents may be clinically more appropriate in different clinical circumstances. Onset times indicate an average time to onset of surgical anaesthesia and duration times signify the likely duration of an accurately placed block.

Section 4, 'Reference', has been incorporated for the benefit of those wishing to read more widely around the subject. The sections of the body have been listed in a similar manner to Sections 2 and 3, and we have used popular regional anaesthesia textbook and journal sources to provide the reference material.

H.B.J. Fischer
C.A. Pinnock   Redditch, 2004

Acknowledgements

The authors would like to thank Carl Young for acting as the model of the photographs, Dr Robert Jones for some original line diagrams and Dr Monica Hardwick, Consultant Anaesthetist, Worcestershire Acute Hospitals Trust, for writing the section on ophthalmic surgery.

Smiths Medical generously supported the cost of colour photography throughout sections 2 and 3.

Contents

Indications for central neuraxial blockade 141

Techniques of central neuraxial blocks 143

Section 4   Appendix

Drug nomenclature

Throughout this volume, the International Non-Proprietary Name (INN) convention of the World Health Organisation (WHO) has been applied. Alternative names for drugs that are referred to frequently within the book are listed below:

Figure 1.1
Drug nomenclature and alternative names

INN	Alternative name
Bupivacaine	Marcaine, Sensorcaine,
Levo bupivacaine	Chirocaine
Ropivacaine	Naropin
Lidocaine	Xylocaine, lignocaine
Prilocaine	Citanest
2-Chloroprocaine	Nesacaine
Mepivacaine	Carbocaine
Tetracaine	Amethocaine
Epinephrine	Adrenaline
Norepinephrine	Noradrenaline
Clonidine	Catapres
Fentanyl	Sublimaze
Midazolam	Hypnovel

Section 1

Principles and practice

Benefits of regional anaesthesia

How to use regional anaesthesia

Regional anaesthesia equipment

Complications of regional anaesthesia

Pharmacology of local anaesthetic drugs

Benefits of regional anaesthesia

Quality of analgesia

Local anaesthetic agents reversibly inhibit sodium ion conductance through specific sodium channels present in the cell membranes of the nervous system. This prevents the transmission of noxious stimuli via the peripheral and central nervous systems to the brain. This prevention of nociception distinguishes regional anaesthesia from all other systemically acting analgesic drugs, which can only modulate the responses of the pain pathway after the stimulus has occurred. The quality of analgesia available with regional anaesthesia is unsurpassed and particularly well suited to peri-operative and acute pain management.

Other categories of analgesic drugs are used in conjunction with local anaesthetic drugs to provide adjuvant analgesia, either in combination with the local anaesthetic injection or separately by systemic administration to provide *balanced* or *multi-modal analgesia*. Non-steroidal anti-inflammatory drugs (NSAIDs) inhibit the sensitisation of peripheral pain receptors and opioids, alpha-2 agonists and other receptor agonists/antagonists modulate the perception of pain at a central level by altering the activity of specific nociceptive receptors within the spinal cord. By combining different analgesic modalities, the quality and duration of analgesia are improved using lower concentrations and volumes of local anaesthetic drugs, compared to using the local anaesthetic as the sole agent. In most cases, the combination of drugs acts synergistically rather than purely summatively.

Duration of analgesia

Analgesia for acute pain, whether following surgery, trauma or other causes, will be necessary for a variable period of time, depending on the severity of the underlying cause. A single bolus injection can provide analgesia from just a few hours up to two days by varying the choice of regional anaesthetic technique, the local anaesthetic used, the concentration and volume injected. For more prolonged analgesia a continuous infusion can be used, both centrally and peripherally. Major thoracic or abdominal surgery requires prolonged post-operative analgesia and a bolus thoracic or lumbar epidural used to establish surgical quality analgesia for the operation can be followed with a continuous post-operative infusion for several days. As the intensity of the pain diminishes, so the infusion rate can be reduced to match the patient's requirements. Many intermediate and minor surgical procedures have a relatively short duration of severe post-operative pain for which a few hours of intense analgesia are all that may be necessary. Day case procedures fall into this category and respond well to peripheral nerve blocks of 3–6 h duration enabling the patient to be discharged pain free without the risks associated with prolonged motor, sensory and proprioceptive dysfunction. Short-acting spinal and epidural blocks are increasingly used for day case surgery, offering excellent surgical anaesthesia and early post-operative analgesia whilst still allowing early discharge from hospital compared to general anaesthesia. For major upper and lower limb surgery, effective analgesia of 12 h or more is possible when the brachial plexus or the sciatic and femoral nerves are blocked with bupivacaine 0.5%. Bupivacaine 0.75% will produce over 24 h analgesia when used to block the femoral and sciatic nerves for major lower limb surgery.

Insertion of epidural, spinal and peripheral nerve catheters can extend the duration of a block over several days by using either intermittent bolus injections or a continuous infusion. Continuous infusions provide an equal quality of analgesia compared to intermittent bolus administration but may use a larger total volume of drug over the course of the infusion. There is less need for intervention by nursing or medical staff with a continuous infusion, although occasional 'top-up' boluses may be required to prevent regression of the block level.

Patient-controlled central and peripheral regional block infusions are increasingly popular with a reduction in hourly drug volume usage and good quality analgesia obtainable. Peripheral patient-controlled analgesia (PCA) techniques have even been used following day case surgery, patients being sent home with wound instillation or peripheral nerve block catheters for up to 48 h.

Peri-operative use

Pain that occurs prior to surgery can be debilitating and can complicate the management of the patient. Ischaemic, trauma or inflammatory pain can have a major impact on patient well being and can be difficult to treat effectively because such pain tends to be opioid resistant. Many patients with ischaemic lower limb pain suffer from diabetes mellitus and the presence of pain (often complicated by infection) can destabilise insulin requirements. The use of large doses of opioids will often compound the problems and in this situation the pre-operative use of an epidural infusion or femoral and sciatic blockade (with catheters inserted into the nerve sheaths if possible) removes the need for opioid drugs and can simplify diabetic management. The pre-operative use of either central neural blockade or peripheral nerve blocks to abolish severe acute pain prior to surgery is of considerable interest as it may influence how pain is perceived post-operatively. There is some evidence that the peri-operative use of regional anaesthesia techniques can prevent the 'chronification' of pain in thoracic surgery (post-thoracotomy syndrome) and in patients undergoing amputation. The latter are likely to suffer from phantom limb pain post-operatively (up to 90% incidence in the first year) and the severity of the pain usually reflects the intensity of the pain experienced pre-operatively. The effective management of pain in the peri-operative period is therefore not only justifiable on humanitarian grounds but may well have a longer-term benefit in preventing or reducing the likelihood of chronic pain problems.

Autonomic neural blockade

In addition to somatic sensory and motor block, regional anaesthesia also produces autonomic neural blockade, which is beneficial both in pain management and in maintaining optimal peripheral vascular circulation. Blockade of the spinal sympathetic chain or the autonomic nerves that accompany the major peripheral plexuses and nerves, produces peripheral vasodilatation proportional to the extent of the autonomic blockade. This effect is of value in the diagnosis and treatment of peripheral vascular disease, producing an improvement in blood flow to areas of critical perfusion. Prolonged vasodilatation also produces improved graft survival in vascular surgical procedures. Brachial plexus anaesthesia produces vasodilatation and improved perfusion in the upper limb and is indicated for trauma surgery (although the risk of obscuring compartment syndrome must be borne in mind), plastic and reconstructive surgery and the fashioning of arterio-venous fistulae.

There is increasing evidence that a number of chronic pain syndromes, especially complex regional pain syndrome, have a degree of sympathetically maintained pain caused by autonomic nervous system dysfunction. Prolonged regional anaesthesia infusions, either central or peripheral, can abolish the pain and allow rehabilitation of the affected limb or joint over a number of days.

Outcome benefits

The benefits of regional anaesthesia are not simply due to the relief of pain at the site of injury. The systemic effects of pain are widespread (Figure 1.1) and the consequences

Figure 1.1
Systemic effects of pain

System	Response to pain
Cardiovascular	↑ Catecholamine release ↑ Myocardial oxygen demand ↑ Myocardial contractility Tachycardia Hypertension ↑ Risk of thrombo-embolic events
Respiratory	↓ Vital capacity ↓ Functional residual capacity ↓ Tidal volume ↓ Peak expiratory flow rate Impaired coughing ↑ Risk of chest infection
Gastro-intestinal	↓ Organ perfusion ↑ Secretions ↑ Sphincter tone ↓ Motility (ileus) Gastric dilatation ↑ Risk of nausea and vomiting
Renal	Sodium and water retention Potassium loss Urinary retention
Metabolism	↑ Catabolic effects Weight loss (lean muscle mass) Disturbed sleep Fatigue

Figure 1.2
The stress response to surgery

1. ↑ Catabolism	↑ Catecholamines, glucagons, growth hormone, ADH, cortisol, renin
2. ↓ Anabolism	↑ Insulin resistance → Hyperglycaemia ↓ Testosterone and insulin secretion ↑ Nitrogen losses → Hypoproteinaemia ↑ Lipolysis and oxidation
3. Fluid balance	↑ Sodium and water retention Hypokalaemia
4. Clinical effects	Weight loss, sleep disturbance, fatigue increased risk of morbidity/mortality

of its ineffective management are manifested in an increased risk of post-operative complications, slower recovery, delayed discharge and increased mortality. The systemic stress response (Figure 1.2) may be triggered by severe pain resulting from any cause and is responsible for some of the adverse outcome from surgery.

Over the last three decades there has been intense speculation and detailed research into the influence of different anaesthetic techniques on the stress response. It is now widely accepted that the complex neuro-endocrine, metabolic and immunological changes that occur after surgery have a detrimental effect on the cardiovascular system, the respiratory system and the gastro-intestinal tract. Many studies have shown that neural blockade with local anaesthetic agents can be effective in abolishing the stress response. The relationship between good analgesia, the abolition of the stress response and a measurable improvement in outcome is complex and there is a lack of data from well-conducted randomised trials because of insufficient numbers in even the largest trials. To detect a significant difference in a rare but important outcome parameter, such as mortality, very large numbers of patients need to be recruited, well beyond what is possible for a single study. The consensus is that properly managed regional anaesthetic techniques are the most effective way of providing post-operative analgesia for major surgery and offer the best available means of modifying the stress response to surgery and of improving outcome. A systematic review by the CORTRA group (Collaborative Overview of Randomised Trials of Regional Anaesthesia) has confirmed that both spinal and epidural anaesthesia have a consistent advantage over general anaesthesia in outcome from surgery. Patients who receive a spinal or an epidural, either as the sole anaesthetic technique or in combination with a general anaesthetic, suffer less morbidity from cardiovascular, respiratory, gastro-intestinal and infective complications and as a result there is a 30% reduction in the risk of death, compared to general anaesthesia alone.

How to use regional anaesthesia

Introduction

In the initial stages of learning about regional anaesthesia the emphasis is justifiably concentrated on practical competency, acquiring the skills necessary for safe and successful block performance. Early success generates further enthusiasm to practice newly acquired skills and learn a greater variety of techniques. Eventually, these skills need to be incorporated into clinical practice to the overall benefit of the patient. Experience is required to select the most appropriate technique (or combination of techniques), to decide whether to use the technique(s) alone or in combination with intravenous sedation or general anaesthesia and to learn how to manage a patient undergoing surgery 'under local'. If the potential benefits of regional anaesthesia are to be fully realised, it is important to realise that injecting the local anaesthetic drug and confirming that the block is working mark only the beginning of the patient's care. Managing the regional block during surgery requires organisation and attention in detail, especially if the patient remains conscious and is not going to regret staying awake during their operation.

Anatomical principles

It is vital to have a proper knowledge of the relevant topographical landmarks for the proposed regional technique and to fully appreciate the anatomical relationships of the intervening structures between the skin and the target nerve(s).

Central neural techniques

The anatomy of the thoracic spine, the lumbar spine and the sacrum, including the ligaments and other soft tissue structures that make up the spinal column is essential information. Each segmental pair of spinal nerves has a symmetrical distribution and typically each spinal nerve has a cutaneous innervation (except C1), somatic sensory distribution to deep structures and motor innervation to a defined muscle group. Some spinal nerves continue peripherally as single nerves (such as

the intercostal nerves) but many combine with adjacent spinal nerves to form complex plexuses (brachial, lumbar and sacral). The cutaneous sensory distribution of the spinal nerves is traditionally shown as a dermatomal map (Figure 1.3) and the innervation of deeper structures is similarly represented by myotomal and osteotomal maps.

Peripheral neural techniques

A typical peripheral nerve will have a cutaneous sensory component, a somatic component supplying motor fibres to muscles and sensory and proprioceptive fibres to joints and other deep structures. The composition of each nerve will vary according to the constituent nerve roots, which combine to form the nerve, some

Figure 1.3
Dermatomal map of spinal nerve distribution

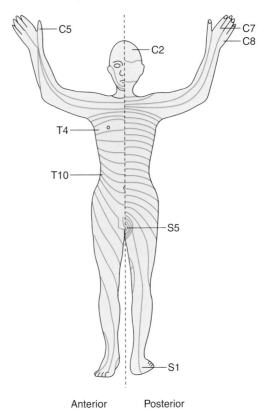

nerves becoming entirely sensory in function and some purely motor. It is possible to construct a map of the dermatomal, myotomal and osteotomal supply for each nerve. For a peripheral nerve with mixed nerve root origins, the cutaneous sensory territory is different to the dermatomal distribution of its constituent nerve roots because an individual dermatome represents a single nerve root whereas the peripheral nerve territory is derived from multiple nerve roots.

If a local anaesthetic block is performed at the level of the nerve roots (such as a thoracic paravertebral or an interscalene brachial plexus block), the onset of anaesthesia occurs in a dermatomal distribution and any inadequacy will show as a dermatomal pattern. If the block is performed more distally (at the level of plexus trunk or a peripheral nerve) then failure will occur in the distribution of one or more nerve territories. Knowledge of the limits of both dermatomes and individual nerve territories is therefore necessary when planning peripheral nerve blocks.

The cutaneous nerve supply to an area does not necessarily correspond to the nerve supply to the underlying structures. The musculo-cutaneous nerve (C5, 6, 7) supplies the flexor muscles in the upper arm but its cutaneous distribution is in the forearm (the lateral cutaneous nerve of forearm). It is important to understand the significance of these differences between the motor and sensory components of a nerve block because they can be utilised during surgery. For instance, surgery for Dupuytren's contracture can be undertaken by blocking the ulnar and median nerves at the wrist, which produces sensory block in the surgical field while the motor supply to the forearm muscles remains unaffected. The surgeon can then ask the patient to move the fingers and help identify the flexor tendons during the surgery.

Hilton's law: The motor nerve to a muscle tends to supply a sensory branch to the joint that the muscle moves and another branch to the skin over the joint. This principle is important in planning procedures for joint surgery. In the knee, for example, the sensory innervation of the intra-articular structures derives from the obturator, femoral, sciatic and lateral cutaneous nerve of thigh which need to be blocked in varying combinations, depending on the type of surgery planned for the knee.

Surgical principles

Part of the planning process for a regional anaesthetic technique includes a clear under-standing of the surgeon's intentions. In turn, the surgeon must understand the constraints that regional anaesthesia imposes on the surgical procedure and be prepared to modify the surgical technique if necessary. Surgery within the thoracic or upper abdominal cavity under a central neural blockade (CNB) is not really practicable and would normally require a general anaesthetic to be included as part of the anaesthetic technique. The surgical procedure will not be unduly affected by the presence of a functioning thoracic or lumbar epidural. Lower abdominal surgery is commonly performed under spinal, epidural or combined spinal and epidural anaesthesia and although the block may be extensive and intense, should the surgeon stimulate structures that are innervated by nerves not blocked by the regional technique, the patient will experience pain or other noxious stimuli. This can occur when abdominal packs are inserted high in the abdomen or visceral organs are placed under tension so that the peritoneum is stretched above the upper limit of the block. Careful handling of organs with minimal blunt dissection and gentle placement of packs and retractors will minimise the likelihood of such reflex pain.

For body surface and limb surgery the following factors must be considered.

- The site of the surgical incision may cross the territory of several adjacent nerves. Even if the incision is entirely within the normal territory of a single nerve, it is prudent to block adjacent nerve territories as there may be considerable variation and overlap. The operation may also turn out to be more extensive than first planned.
- Surgery above the knee or elbow usually requires plexus anaesthesia whereas surgery distal to the elbow or knee can be undertaken using discrete nerve blocks. However, even for distal surgery, a tourniquet may be required and a plexus block will be necessary so that the patient can tolerate the tourniquet.
- Surgical stimulation may cause the patient distress despite a functioning somatic block. Traction on the spermatic cord can occur during hernia or scrotal surgery and produce visceral pain in the abdomen. It is vital that the surgeon is fully aware of the limitations

of regional anaesthesia in this situation and modifies the surgical technique accordingly.

Patient selection

Successful regional anaesthesia requires active co-operation and involvement from the patient who, in turn, can expect to be fully informed about the process by the anaesthetist concerned.

Informed consent

This is an essential pre-requisite for all local and regional anaesthesia techniques. For most patients a brief outline of the intended technique and its benefits (quality and duration of the pain relief, reduction in nausea, vomiting, drowsiness, earlier return to oral fluids and food, etc.) usually results in a willing patient. Benefits need to be balanced by a discussion of the common side effects and complications of the intended technique. The extent to which side effects and complications are discussed depends on the likely incidence with which they occur balanced against their potential severity. For example, post-dural puncture headache with an incidence of approximately 1% may need to be discussed in relation to an epidural block, even though its sequelae are not life threatening. Whereas major permanent neurological damage need not be discussed because its incidence is so small (<1; 10,000), even though its effects on the patient may be very severe. However, if a patient asks a direct question about a particular aspect of the process then an honest and balanced answer should be given. Specific, written consent is not necessary although a note should be made on the patient's anaesthetic chart that the discussion took place and the patient consented. Consent is designed to inform, not frighten and the precise details need to be tailored to the individual's needs and understanding for the use of a particular technique. No patient should be coerced into a regional technique against his or her will but where the risk benefit ratio is clearly in favour of regional anaesthesia, this should be pointed out to the patient before accepting their refusal to undergo regional anaesthesia.

In some patient groups co-operation may not be possible and regional anaesthesia may need to be supplemented with intravenous sedation or general anaesthesia. Many patients who are reluctant to accept the concept of remaining awake whilst undergoing surgery are happy to co-operate if they know that sedation or anaesthesia is possible. Children present specific problems. The older child may well co-operate, especially if local anaesthetic cream is used to make skin penetration painless but for those too frightened or too young to understand the procedure, general anaesthesia will be necessary prior to the local block.

The preparation of a patient for major surgery under regional anaesthesia is similar to that for general anaesthesia. If the patient is not fit for general anaesthesia then a regional technique is not necessarily going to be a suitable alternative. Appropriate clinical, laboratory and radiological data should be available and any pathophysiological disturbance should be investigated and treated before instituting regional anaesthesia which must not be regarded as a 'short cut' or less demanding alternative to general anaesthesia.

Contraindications to regional anaesthesia

There are relatively few absolute contraindications to either central or peripheral nerve blockade. Relative contraindications can be assessed on an individual basis and the benefits balanced against the risk. By modifying patient treatment or the intended regional technique, regional anaesthesia can often be used with minimum risk even in the presence of some of the contraindications listed in Figure 1.4. For instance, infection or trauma over the site of the proposed block may prevent one technique but a more proximal or distal combination of blocks is often possible.

Figure 1.4
Contraindications to regional anaesthesia

- Patient refusal despite adequate explanation
- Psychiatric or psychological disturbance
- Unco-operative patient (aggression, fear, restlessness)
- Systemic infections
- Trauma or infection over site of injection
- Coagulopathy or full anticoagulation
- Chronic neurological disease (especially demyelinating disease)
- Untreated hypovolaemia (particularly central neural blocks)
- Raised intracranial pressure (central neural blocks)

Bacterial infection

Sepsis or bacteraemia is not a contraindication to peripheral nerve blocks unless there is a septic focus directly involving the site of skin puncture or the perineural tissues of the proposed block. Not only will this increase the risk of morbidity from the injection but the block is also unlikely to be effective, as the acid pH of the surrounding tissue will inactivate the local anaesthetic drug. An alternative site for the peripheral nerve block, either proximal or distal to the site of infection, may be possible with careful consideration of the site of surgery and the appropriate nerve supply.

CNB, both spinal and epidural, is contraindicated where there is evidence of active systemic infection because of the serious risk of haematogenous or direct spread of infection into the epidural space or the cerebrospinal fluid (CSF). If an epidural or a spinal is strongly indicated, and time allows, they may be considered if blood cultures prove negative and the patient has received an adequate course of the appropriate antibiotic.

Areas of chronically inflamed or diseased skin (psoriasis, eczema, hydradinitis, etc.) are also best avoided for the site of the puncture.

Viral infection

Acute episodes of herpes simplex can produce significant viraemia and regional anaesthesia is probably best avoided during this phase of the infection, although once the lesion is localised, peripheral nerve blocks are not thought to be a risk factor.

Patients with acquired immune deficiency syndrome (AIDS) caused by the human immunodeficiency virus (HIV) virus may present with serious associated systemic disease and be ideally suited to the use of regional anaesthesia. However, in addition to the increased concerns about invasive procedures in such patients and the increased risks of needlestick injury, there are also concerns about HIV damage to neurological tissue. The HIV virus causes demyelination of the central nervous system and therefore regional anaesthesia should be considered a contraindication in patients with evidence of peripheral neuropathy or altered central neural responses.

Neurological disease

Local anaesthetic drugs can accelerate the process of demyelination within the central nervous system and therefore regional anaesthesia techniques should be avoided in patients with active demyelinating conditions such as Guillan–Barré syndrome, amyotrophic sclerosis and probably in the relapsing phases of multiple sclerosis. All patients must be considered on the merits of the block for each individual and there may be circumstances where CNB is appropriate for a particular patient's needs. In patients with multiple sclerosis, which is currently stable or quiescent, full discussion with the patient is essential, if regional anaesthesia is contemplated as there may well be a temporary worsening of the patient's symptoms in the post-operative course. This pattern of temporary deterioration is common after surgery even without regional anaesthesia and patients need to aware of this.

Peripheral neuropathy is less of a problem and in conditions such as diabetic neuropathy, regional anaesthesia may well be the technique of choice for peripheral limb or body surface surgery. However, the risk benefit analysis should be documented in favour of regional anaesthesia in case of a change in post-operative nerve function.

If a patient has had a previous cerebro-vascular accident (CVA), careful consideration must be given to the timing of the CVA and whether it was embolic or haemorrhagic. After a period of 6 months, there should be minimal risk in using a spinal or epidural with an old CVA provided that motor and sensory function has stabilised. Where the stroke is recent, particularly if haemorrhagic, regional anaesthesia is probably contraindicated. This applies particularly to patients receiving treatment that alters their blood coagulation.

Coagulopathy

Altered coagulation status can arise from pre-existing liver or haematological disease and from the administration of anticoagulation therapy. Anticoagulant therapy may be necessary for pre-existing disease states (atrial fibrillation, thromboembolic episodes and prosthetic heart valves) or may be used during the peri-operative period for antithrombotic prophylaxis. Each patient's requirements will vary; if time allows and their surgical condition warrants regional anaesthesia, it may be possible to manipulate the anticoagulant therapy so that regional anaesthesia does not cause undue risk. For example, patients awaiting elective orthopaedic surgery can be instructed to stop taking drugs such as aspirin or non-steroidal anti-inflammatory drugs (NSAIDs) 3–10 days prior to surgery (see Figure 1.6). Prothrombin time (PT), or its standardised equivalent, the International Normalised Ratio (INR), and activated partial thromboplastin time (APTT) are the best routine indicators of the integrity of the extrinsic and intrinsic coagulation systems and give a good overall idea of the state of coagulation. However there is no satisfactory routine test for platelet function and patient history and examination for signs of excessive bruising or easy bleeding is also important.

The major risks of regional anaesthesia in the presence of altered coagulation are the creation of a compressive haematoma or neural ischaemia, particularly within the spinal canal. Spinal haematoma remains a very rare but serious complication despite the increased use of thromboembolic prophylaxis. However, the introduction of low molecular weight heparin (LMWH) in the USA during the 1990s produced an increased number of case reports of spinal haematoma, mainly due to the large doses recommended for prophylaxis and also the timing of the administration. As a result, the American Society of Regional Anaesthesia produced a Consensus Statement on the use of thromboembolic prophylaxis with regional anaesthesia and more recently the European Society of Regional Anaesthesia has produced *Clinical Practice Guidelines for Thromboprophylaxis and Central Neural Blockade* (Figure 1.5).

Central neural blocks are known to reduce the incidence of peri-operative thromboembolic disease in major surgery and therefore reduce morbidity and mortality. Their use, together with other devices such as antiembolism stockings, sequential pneumatic compression of the lower limbs and active mobilisation may be sufficient to delay the need for unfractionated heparin (UFH) or LMWH until after the block has been established.

Patient management

Pre-operative management

It is essential to communicate effectively with the patient throughout the conduct of the

regional anaesthesia and surgery. Each stage of block performance and management needs to be discussed with the patient. Whilst complications are rare and largely avoidable, common side effects such as motor, autonomic and proprioceptive dysfunction may worry the patient unless they are discussed in advance. Minor side effects such as stinging from the initial injection of the local anaesthetic solution or the paraesthesiae that accompany the onset and offset of the block need to be addressed. The possibility of motor weakness outlasting the return of sensation should be emphasised and pain management after the block has worn off needs also to be discussed.

The patient may experience a variety of sensations during surgery despite a fully functioning block and this needs to be fully explained to prevent them being interpreted as a sign of failed anaesthesia. These non-specific sensations (pressure, tissue tension and disordered temperature sensation) are common and may be disconcerting. These feelings should not cause distress but need to be discussed as the patient may interpret them as painful even when they are not. Reassurance that this is normal and not a sign of a failed technique is necessary to maintain patient confidence. It is important to explain to the patient the likely effects of the motor and sensory loss that will last into the post-operative period. This avoids the patient misinterpreting the apparent loss of part of their anatomy during their early post-operative recovery. Some patients become distressed by the apparent loss of part of their body (perhaps reflecting lack of central body image recognition) and need reassurance to deal with this abnormal sensation – often until the block has completely regressed.

The decision about whether to use regional anaesthesia alone or to combine it with general anaesthesia must be decided at the pre-operative visit and fully explored. Light general anaesthesia is easier and safer to manage than several boluses of intravenous sedation, which may become necessary during surgery if the patient becomes unco-operative. Recovery from a light inhalational general anaesthetic or a total intravenous anaesthetic is quicker and more predictable than from intravenous benzodiazepine sedation, which can be accompanied by marked post-operative sedation.

Figure 1.5
The European Society of Regional Anaesthesia (ESRA) *Clinical Practice Guidelines for Thromboprophylaxis and Central Neural Blockade*

- Maximum probable incidence of spinal haematoma following CNB in patients without risk factors:
  - 1:320,000 for spinals,
  - 1:190,000–200,000 for epidurals.
- Maximum risk occurs with epidural catheterisation.
- Minimum risk occurs with single shot narrow gauge spinal needle.
- 60–80% of significant bleeds associated with bloody taps or clotting disorders.
- 30–60% bleeds occur on removal of catheter.

Risk factors

Patient factors	Technique factors
Spinal abnormality	Technical difficulty
Age > 70 year	Repeated attempts
Female	Traumatic puncture
Anticoagulant therapy	Use of catheter
Existing coagulopathy	Catheter removal

Unfractionated heparin (UFH)

- *Prophylactic doses*: very extensive experience with UFH. No appreciable increase in risk if:
  - interval of 4 h between a dose of 5000 units of UFH and insertion or removal of catheter or
  - 1 h interval after insertion of needle or removal of catheter before next dose of UFH administered.
- Beware of concurrent therapy that may also alter coagulation status.
- No monitoring required for 4 days. After this platelet counts are mandatory because of risk of heparin-induced thrombocytopenia (HIT).
- *Therapeutic doses*: for vascular or cardiac surgery. Start injections/infusions 1 h after needle/catheter placement and maintain partial thromboplastin time (PTT) at 1.5 times normal. Remove catheter 4 h after stopping infusion and check that PTT, activated clotting time (ACT) and platelet count are normal.

Low molecular weight heparin (LMWH)

- *Prophylaxis*: no increased risk compared to UFH with up to 40 mg/day of enoxaparin (or equivalent), provided that there are no additional risk factors and there is a 10–12 h interval between last dose of LMWH and either needle placement or catheter removal. There should be a 6–8 h interval then before the next dose of LMWH and therefore a once daily dosing regimen is preferable.

Antiplatelet agents

- Very little evidence of problems in the absence of other risk factors
- Beware the use of concurrent therapy – dextrans, anticoagulants, heparin
- If time allows, stop therapy 1–3 days pre-operatively for NSAIDs and >3 days for aspirin, ticlopidine and other antiplatelet drugs
- Otherwise, measure platelets, careful visual inspection for signs of disordered coagulation plus bleeding history. There are no universally accepted tests for adequate platelet function.

Oral anticoagulants

- Therapeutic levels of coumarins are an absolute contraindication
- Stop agent, convert to heparin, and monitor INR, PT and APTT (factor VII, but also factors II and X affected)
- If INR < 1.5 proceed with caution (spinal rather than epidural)
- Beware catheter removal

Figure 1.6
Indications for combining general and regional anaesthesia

- Patient preference
- Surgical technique – if surgery causes reflex stimuli outside area of anaesthesia, for example traction on spermatic cord during herniorraphy under field block
- Prolonged operation – beyond 1 h, many patients find it very uncomfortable to lie still
- Tourniquet pain
- Amputations
- Cancer surgery

Indications for combining general and regional anaesthesia are listed in Figure 1.6.

Premedication

The use of premedication for patients undergoing regional anaesthesia is subject to the same guidelines that apply to general anaesthesia. Many patients are happy to avoid any sedation and clouding of consciousness following an adequate explanation of what to expect, whilst others prefer to know little of the actual surgery. Much will depend on the skills and confidence of the person performing the technique. Where premedication is prescribed, the patient must remain able to co-operate during the regional technique, therefore heavy sedation should be avoided.

Pre-operative starvation

A patient who is to receive regional anaesthesia should undergo the same protocol of pre-operative restriction of fluids and food as patients undergoing the same procedure under general anaesthesia. Sudden loss of consciousness can occur for a number of reasons during the conduct of regional anaesthesia. The patient is therefore exposed to the same risks of regurgitation or vomiting as during general anaesthesia. Starvation is essential in the event that inadequate anaesthesia requires supplementation with general anaesthesia.

Performing the technique

All regional techniques are capable of causing complications. Local anaesthetic drugs have potentially serious toxic properties. No patient should undergo regional anaesthesia unless the operator is fully trained in the recognition of complications and is competent to treat them. Full resuscitation facilities must be immediately available together with suitable patient monitoring equipment.

Safe conduct of regional anaesthesia requires suitable surroundings of cleanliness and space with a good source of ambient light and warmth with adequate privacy for the patient. An assistant trained in anaesthesia and recovery procedures and familiar with regional anaesthesia must be available to assist both doctor and the patient. If the patient is comfortable and correctly positioned and the operator is comfortable and well prepared, then the chances of the technique being performed quickly and successfully is increased. The equipment, sterile towels and drugs required for the procedure should be available and checked before the patient is positioned. The bed or trolley should be adjusted to the correct height for the operator and the patient positioned comfortably and accurately, using pillows and other supports as indicated. The assistant can help the patient to maintain the correct position and will often provide psychological support and reassurance, allowing the clinician to concentrate on the procedure. Once the technique is started, conversation should be restricted to informing the patient as to what to expect next with reassurance as necessary. If an explanation of the technique is being given to observers, then the patient must be informed so that they do not misinterpret remarks. Explanations given in the presence of a conscious patient must take into account the patient's situation and understanding.

Where local anaesthesia is to be combined with a general anaesthesia, some authorities advocate performing the blocks with the patient awake on the grounds of avoiding inadvertent intraneural injection. However, the majority of children receive their local anaesthetic block after induction of general anaesthesia without evidence of an increased risk of neural damage. In adults many techniques such as intercostal, interpleural, caudal, femoral and sciatic nerve blocks are traditionally performed after induction of anaesthesia without demonstrable extra risk. Provided that appropriate care is taken to avoid intraneural and intravascular injection, most regional techniques can be performed

Figure 1.7
The Bromage motor block scale

THE BROMAGE MOTOR BLOCK SCALE (1965)		
Degree of motor block	**Bromage criterion**	**Score (%)**
1. No block	Full flexion of knees and feet	0
2. Partial block	Just able to flex knees plus full flexion of feet	33
3. Almost complete	Unable to flex knees, some foot flexion still	66
4. Complete	Unable to move legs or feet	100

under general anaesthesia if necessary. Epidural injections above the cauda equina and the interscalene approach to the brachial plexus are safer performed in conscious patients.

Testing the block

Both the motor and sensory components of a block must be tested during the onset of the block. This will monitor the rate of onset of the block and the ultimate extent of the block. The sensory loss is tested either with pinprick (using a blunted neurological examination needle) or loss of cold perception to ice. Finger pressure touch and pinching of the skin are also used to confirm sensory loss over the operative site. Motor loss can be graded using the original or modified Bromage scale (Figure 1.7) for central neural blocks or the loss of muscle power in flexion and extension for peripheral nerve blocks. Although dermatomal loss of sensation will define the upper and lower levels of cutaneous sensory block, loss of sensation of superficial and deep structures in the region of the operative site (myotomes and osteotomes) may not reflect this. Where possible, separate testing of the deeper structures response to pressure should also be performed. The ultimate test is successful completion of the operation without patient discomfort.

Peri-operative management

The operating theatre can appear to be a hostile and intimidating environment to the conscious patient and all staff should be aware of the noise and other disturbances they make. Every step of the preparation and positioning of the patient

should be explained and directed towards making them comfortable and confident. On no account should any preparations for surgery begin until the patient is confident in the quality of the anaesthesia. Resist the temptation to repeatedly question the patient as to what they can feel. Explain to them what to expect as the block develops, ask them to say when the different stages happen and use objective tests of motor and sensory loss in the area of the block to decide on the adequacy of the analgesia. Dissuade the surgeon from saying 'Can you feel this?' or 'Does this hurt?' as they make the incision. Remind the patient of the sensations that were discussed during the pre-operative visit.

If significant motor weakness occurs, the affected part must be properly protected from hyperextension injury due to unrestrained movement and all the relevant pressure points must be well protected during surgery. Once the operation is underway and much of the noise of preparation subsides, many patients will drift off to sleep if they are comfortable and have been premedicated or if a small dose of intravenous sedation is used. Others prefer to have a gentle conversation or even watch their procedure on screen, which the increasing use of video technology makes possible.

Documenting the block

There is a mandatory requirement to record all the important facts relating to the performance and management of a block. The amount of information recorded will vary according to the complexity of the block but the minimum dataset for all major techniques should include the parameters listed in Figure 1.8.

Figure 1.8
The regional anaesthetic record

- Named technique and approach
- Type of needle
- Use of nerve stimulator (or not) and minimum current used (mA)
- Use of catheter
- The agent, its concentration and volume (including vasoconstrictor or other additives)
- Onset times for motor and sensory block (bilateral or unilateral)
- Extent of dermatomal block and degree of motor block
- The occurrence of any paraesthesiae or pain on needle or catheter insertion
- Bleeding or other sequelae of the injection should also be noted

Post-operative care

Short-stay surgery

The degree of supervision required post-operatively depends on the anticipated duration and the extent of the block. For day case, outpatient and emergency department surgery the prime requirement is early mobilisation and discharge with the patient able to self-care. To achieve this, nerve blockade should be as peripheral as possible and of short duration rather than central or proximal peripheral blocks of long duration. There are inherent risks associated with flail limbs – the arm is an important part of balance and self-protection and the leg is essential for weight bearing. The patient should not be discharged until the motor block has fully regressed. If for any reason a limb is still affected by a block at the time of discharge, it should either be immobilised in a sling for protection or the patient must remain non-weight bearing during the journey home and instructed to rest until full function returns.

Inpatient surgery

For major surgery, long duration of analgesia is a benefit, provided that due regard is paid to the specific care of the anaesthetised area. CNB can produce widespread sensory, motor and autonomic effects that require specific monitoring throughout their duration of action. Pain charts should also chart the regression of block height and motor weakness in addition to measuring pain scores and haemodynamic values. If opioid-containing infusions are used then respiratory rate and sedation scores must be measured.

Patients who have undergone lower limb blocks or lumbar epidural blockade must only be mobilised under direct supervision until they can demonstrate full motor and sensory recovery. This is tested by the ability to fully flex and extend the hip and knee against resistance (motor) and have normal proprioception and sensation in the great toe (sensory). Some authorities recommend testing perianal skin sensation to ensure complete sacral nerve root recovery but in practice this is not always necessary. The upper limb must be properly immobilised with a sling or other support until full function returns. Any patient who has long-lasting cutaneous analgesia should be encouraged to move the affected limb in order to prevent pressure sores developing on the dependent areas. If the blockade is extensive and intense, nursing and physiotherapy staff must be able to provide regular and frequent postural changes, passive limb movements and pressure relieving aids to prevent dependant pressure damage. Use of lower limb blocks may require antithrombotic precautions until full mobilisation is achieved.

Ischaemic pain

Plaster casts, compression dressings or limb splints can cause vascular inadequacy and ischaemia if incorrectly applied. Early swelling and discolouration should alert attending staff to remove the dressing and examine the limb even though the patient may not complain of pain. Compartment syndrome following closed trauma to a limb can cause major ischaemic damage if unrecognised in the early stages and a functional nerve blockade may delay the awareness of pain until the late stages of ischaemia. Ischaemic pain may break through a block in the same way as pathological pain breaks through functioning epidural blockade but early diagnosis of ischaemic damage is the key to avoiding the later sequelae. All staff involved in the care of patients undergoing regional blockade must understand the implications of prolonged analgesia and modify patient management accordingly. Circulation and skin colour must be assessed at frequent, regular intervals and the results recorded so that any change is noticed quickly and acted upon.

Pain on passive movement of the anaesthetised limb or digit is an early sign of ischaemic pain and again should trigger immediate action. Muscle compartment pressure monitoring can also be used if compartment syndrome is thought to be likely. With appropriate monitoring and management systems in place, regional anaesthesia can be used with benefit in trauma patients or other patient groups at risk, despite the absence of pain sensation.

Sequential analgesia

For many minor and intermediate surgical procedures, a long-acting peripheral nerve block may provide all the analgesia that the patient needs. For more major surgery, a peripheral nerve or plexus infusion or an epidural catheter infusion can maintain the duration of analgesia for several days if necessary. For all but minor operations, pain will outlast the duration of the regional block and it is important to consider the most appropriate means of controlling the pain after the block wears off. A course of compound oral analgesics or non-steroidal anti-inflammatory agents may be sufficient and should be started before the effects of the nerve block wear off completely so that the analgesia remains continuous. For more major surgery, systemic opioid supplementation may be necessary as the regional technique is withdrawn. One or two intramuscular injections of morphine may be all that is necessary to cover the period of transition from an epidural infusion to oral analgesia. Alternatively, intravenous opioid patient-controlled analgesia may be required if pain remains a problem as the regional technique is withdrawn, particularly if technical difficulties mean that the block is discontinued prematurely.

Pain outside the anaesthetised area or breakthrough pain in the immediate post-operative period may need parenteral opioids which can also provide a general sedative effect in patients who have good analgesia but are restless due to other stimuli. It is most important to achieve and maintain good quality analgesia from the outset and to supplement the regional technique as necessary until the patient is comfortable.

Regional anaesthesia equipment

General anaesthesia and resuscitation

All local anaesthetic drugs produce signs and symptoms of cardiovascular and neurological toxicity if an excessive mass of drug is administered or a significant volume is injected intravascularly. Regional anaesthesia demands proficiency at airway management and cardiorespiratory resuscitation and should not be performed without the immediate availability of intravenous therapy, suction, cardiorespiratory resuscitation equipment and monitoring facilities. All personnel involved in patient care during the regional block should be appropriately qualified in basic and preferably advanced life support and facilities for general anaesthesia should be immediately available for back up.

Regional anaesthesia requirements

All techniques should be performed with sterile (preferably disposable) items and the preparation of drugs and equipment should be undertaken in conditions of good light on a surface of adequate size so that sterility can be maintained. The choice of commercially available regional anaesthesia packs or packs produced within the hospital is a matter of local requirements and financial comparisons. There should be sufficient sterile towels of appropriate size to ensure a sterile field; again, the choice of re-usable or disposable sheets is a matter for local choice. Solutions used to sterilise skin should not be replaced on the sterile surface and they must be disposed of before the local anaesthetic solution is drawn up to avoid any potential confusion. The person performing the block should draw up all local anaesthetic drugs and they should be checked with another member of the team before disposal of the ampoules.

Full sterile precautions (face mask, surgical gown and gloves) should be adopted for all central neural blocks and complex peripheral nerve block techniques (such as the placement of catheters). Some authorities are happy that wearing sterile surgical gloves and a facemask after a formal surgical scrubbing of the hands is safe for peripheral blocks in combination with a rigorous no-touch technique.

Needles

Infiltration needles

Fine gauge (23G or 25G) hypodermic needles are used to make preliminary skin wheals of local anaesthetic and are useful for small areas of local anaesthetic infiltration. For infiltration over a wider area, use spinal needles of similar gauge. Twenty-seven gauge needles are useful for children and needle phobic adults.

Central block needles

Spinal needles

Spinal anaesthesia requires specialised needles and introducers in addition to the general equipment necessary for central nerve blocks (Figure 1.9). Spinal needles are available in a

Figure 1.9
Tip design of spinal needles. (a) Euro pencil point, (b) lancet point and (c) pencil point (reproduced with the kind permission of Smiths Medical)

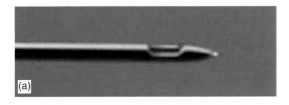

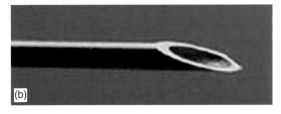

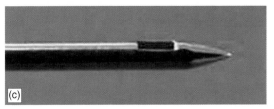

standard shaft length of 8 cm and a range of gauges from 18G to 30G. Shaft lengths of 25–150 mm are available for specialist needs (neonatal, paediatric and very large adults). There is an inevitable incidence of post-dural puncture headache (PDPH) with spinal anaesthesia ranging from 0.2% to 24% and many designs of needle have been introduced to try and reduce this problem. Currently the lowest incidence of PDPH is associated with very narrow gauge, short bevel needles (26–29G) and 24G pencil point, Whitacre tip designs or the more specialised Sprotte designs with a large side-opening hole. The narrow gauge and relatively blunt tips of these needles require insertion through a properly designed introducer, which should be closely matched to the type of spinal needle being used to avoid tip damage.

Epidural needles

The Tuohy needle (Figure 1.10) is the most popular and widely used needle for lumbar and thoracic epidurals, although other designs such as the Crawford and Husted needles are still available. The Tuohy needle has an obturator along its length, which should be checked for a close fitting match to the hub and orifice before using it. Tuohy needles are available in 16–18G and a shaft length of 8–10 cm for adult use. They are also available with wings attached to the hub for additional control of the needle during insertion.

Epidural catheters are introduced through the Tuohy needle once the epidural space is located. They are made of high tensile strength, radio-opaque polyvinylchloride (PVC) and are available in a range of sizes to fit 16–20G Tuohy needles. They combine tensile strength with flexibility as the catheter warms to body temperature and have either one end hole to the catheter or multiple side holes along the last few centimetres. They are usually marked in 1 cm calibrations for the distal 20 cm and the proximal end is fitted with a detachable compression Luerlock fitting for attaching bacterial filters and syringes.

Caudal needles

For adults and large children a 22G short bevel needle is suitable for a single-shot caudal. In babies and small children (under 35 kg) a 23G hypodermic needle is used unless a catheter is to be inserted in which case a 20G

Figure 1.10
Tuohy epidural needle and multi-side hole catheter (reproduced with the kind permission of Smiths Medical)

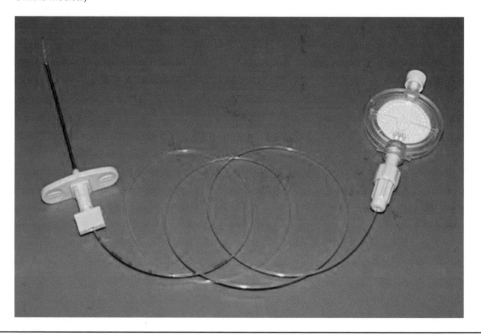

Tuohy needle and catheter are used, although this technique is usually restricted to specialised paediatric units.

Peripheral block needles

Although some minor blocks can be performed with a standard hypodermic needle (penile block, ulnar nerve, webspace blocks, etc.) most discrete nerve blocks are performed with short bevelled needles specifically designed for regional anaesthesia. The bevel angle of standard hypodermic needles is determined by British Standard (BS) No. 5081 Part 2 (1987) with the bevel cut at 12° (with +2/−0° tolerance). They may also be referred to as long bevelled or A bevelled needles. Short, or B bevelled needles have no equivalent BS and the bevel may be cut between 18° and 45°, the facets being ground so that the needle parts tissue rather than cutting it. Short bevel needles offer more resistance during insertion and thus more feedback to the operator. Figure 1.11 shows the overall dimensions and bevel angles of the tip of a typical short bevelled needle. The 'security' bead near the junction of the shaft and the hub was originally necessary to prevent migration and loss of the shaft if the hub broke off due to fatigue of the solder used to join both parts. Modern needles are made from surgical stainless steel with very secure hubs, thus the bead is now redundant although it may be used as an attachment for the alligator clip of a peripheral nerve stimulator (PNS). Short bevelled needles are available from several manufactures in a wide range of shaft lengths and needle gauges. The shaft length varies from 25 to 150 mm and the gauge from 20G to 24G.

There continues to be disagreement and uncertainty about the design of the needle tip and its effect on the incidence of nerve trauma following regional anaesthesia. Selander et al.

(1977) showed that both in vivo and in vitro, short bevel needles cause less damage to nerves and are associated with a lower incidence of neuritis although this view has been challenged by Rice and McMahon (1992) who showed that the reverse was true (albeit in a rat sciatic nerve model). Nevertheless it is clear that there is no clinical data to support the suggestions that needle tip design and the elicitation of paraesthesiae have a direct link with the incidence of neuropathy (Moore et al. 1994). Other research has suggested that needles without any bevel at all would be logical and pencil point needles have been designed to prevent neural damage. Pencil point needles are designed with a side port to prevent intraneural injection, although in a number of studies it has been shown that intraneural as opposed to epineural injection is most unlikely and difficult to reproduce even in vitro.

Despite the controversy surrounding the choice of needle tip, short bevel or pencil point needles are strongly recommended for major nerve blockade because the amount of feedback from them is so superior to long bevelled needles that the likelihood of success is enhanced. The risk of inserting a short bevelled needle into the substance of a peripheral nerve is much less than with a long bevelled one because of the different cutting characteristics of the bevels, although it is accepted that should intraneural placement occur, the damage from the short bevel would be greater than a long bevel.

With the increasing use of peripheral nerve infusions, a variety of perineural infusion catheter kits are available from a number of manufacturers. There are three main categories; cannula over needle, catheter through cannula, Seldinger wire and catheter kits (Figure 1.12). Insulated 18G Tuohy needles are also now available and are useful for some peripheral

Figure 1.11
Regional block needle (reproduced with the kind permission of Smiths Medical)

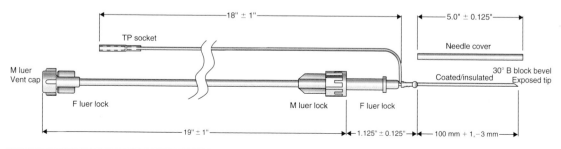

Figure 1.12
A peripheral nerve catheter kit (reproduced with the kind permission of Smiths Medical)

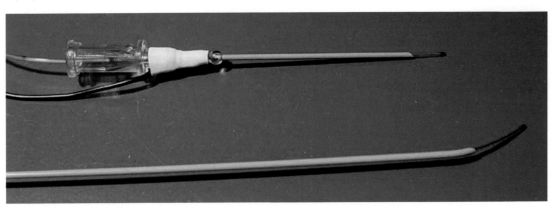

Figure 1.13
Ideal characteristics of a PNS

- Portable, battery operated, with detachable and sterilisable leads
- Clearly marked electrodes indicating that cathode (positive) is attached to needle
- Universal terminals for use with a wide variety of needles
- Digital display of delivered current (and/or voltage) with linear output. Below 1 mA, sensitivity increased to allow precise current readings
- Voltage (9 V) and current (5 mA) limited to cope with variable resistance of body tissues
- Short duration impulse (100–200 ms) at frequency of 1–2 Hz so that motor nerves are stimulated preferentially to sensory nerves

Note: The product of mA and ms is nanocoulombs (nC) and the digital readout of a PNS can be calibrated in nC. For example, 1 mA × 100 ms = 100 nC, which is sufficient charge to stimulate a nerve at a distance of 2–3 mm.

nerve catheter techniques (paravertebral block, femoral block and psoas sheath block).

Peripheral nerve stimulator (PNS)

Low power electrical stimuli have been used to locate peripheral nerves since 1912 but safe, practical and portable PNSs suitable for routine clinical use have only been developed relatively recently. Pither et al. (1984) identified the theoretical electrical characteristics of nerve stimulation and the ideal characteristics for a PNS are well understood (Figure 1.13). There are now some commercially available units that satisfy all theoretical requirements and Figure 1.14 shows the most recent version of a popular model.

Indications

The PNS can stimulate any peripheral nerve of mixed motor and sensory function, typically using a pulse width of 100 ms and a current of <0.5 mA. Purely sensory nerves can be stimulated with a long duration pulse width (>300 ms) at higher power to produce paraesthesiae, although this is an unreliable method and may be uncomfortable for the patient.

The PNS is not a substitute for knowledge of the relevant anatomy and should not be used to hunt blindly for nerves. It is primarily used to confirm accurate placement of a needle tip close to, but not touching the nerve. The PNS is most useful in the location of deeply placed nerves and plexuses, which are traditionally associated with a low success rate when the technique is attempted 'blind'. As each nerve produces a characteristic distribution of muscle movement when stimulated, the PNS may also be appropriate for accurately locating a particular part of a large nerve or plexus when the anaesthetic requirements demand that a specific branch of the nerve be blocked. For example, the deep division of the femoral nerve, which

Figure 1.14
A peripheral nerve stimulator (reproduced with the kind permission of Smiths Medical)

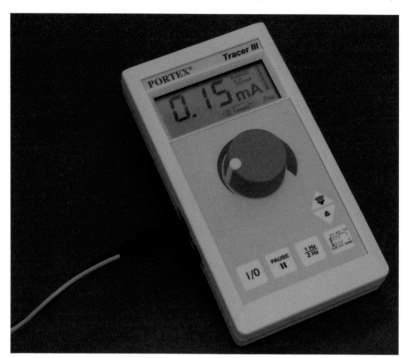

supplies the sensory fibres of the knee joint and the motor supply to the quadriceps femoris and the patellar mechanism, will produce distinct patellar motion, which is not evident, if just the superficial branch is stimulated. The distinct end point of pulse-synchronous muscle movement that accompanies nerve location makes the PNS a valuable aid to learning peripheral nerve blocks and also allows nerve location in patients who are sedated or anaesthetised. The following approaches benefit from the use of a PNS:

- all approaches to brachial plexus
- suprascapular nerve
- radial nerve at the elbow
- median nerve at the elbow
- all approaches to sciatic nerve
- femoral nerve (including '3 in 1')
- obturator nerve
- popliteal fossa block

Using the PNS

1. Connect the anode (positive lead) to a ground electrode. If using an adhesive ECG electrode, ensure that it has a good coating of gel and that it makes good contact with de-greased skin. Place it about 15 cm from the needle insertion point, away from the distribution of the nerve being located.
2. Test the battery power and check circuit integrity (which may be an audible or visual signal depending on the model of PNS).
3. Set the frequency at 1–2 Hz and the delivered current at a moderate level, 2 mA for example.
4. Attach the cathode (negative lead) to the needle electrode and insert the needle towards the nerve, using a standard approach. Turn on the PNS and advance the needle until within the anticipated vicinity of the nerve, carefully observing for any pulse synchronous movement of the muscles.
5. Coulomb's Law (inverse square law) means that the power needed to stimulate a nerve decreases quickly as the distance from needle tip to nerve decreases. With 2 mA or less there will be no pulse synchronous movement until the needle is less than 1 cm from the nerve, unless intervening muscle is directly stimulated by the advancing needle. This is usually easily distinguished from the

distinct pulse synchronous movement of nerve stimulation, seen with current values of 1 mA or less. In order to place the needle tip adjacent to the nerve, carefully adjust the needle tip position whilst reducing the stimulus strength until the muscle movement is just discernible with the minimum stimulus possible (usually 0.3–0.5 mA delivered current). A sudden increase in muscle movement or the onset of pain indicates that the needle is in direct contact with the nerve and it should be withdrawn slightly before the injection. The minimum stimulating current and voltage are affected by a number of factors:

- the nerve being blocked
- the age of the patient
- the presence of neuropathy
- insulated or uninsulated needles

Small, superficial nerves such as the median or radial require only 0.1–0.3 mA while large, deep nerves such as the sciatic or obturator require up to 2 mA. Similarly, greater stimulus strength will be necessary in the elderly compared to young adults and children. Patients with peripheral neuropathy, such as diabetics, also tend to have higher stimulation thresholds. Insulated needles require lower power requirements for nerve stimulation than the equivalent gauge and length of uninsulated needles.

5. Immobilise the needle once the nerve is located and aspirate gently. An initial injection of 1–2 ml may produce an increased muscle movement as the local anaesthetic improves the electrical conductivity but it is quickly followed by a fade in the movement, which is attributed to the nerve being displaced by the injection and thus increasing the needle–nerve distance. Resistance to the flow of injectate or pain on injection indicates subperineural or intraneural needle placement and the injection must be stopped immediately. If the patient is sedated or anaesthetised, pain or paraesthesiae on injection will not be apparent, so extreme care must be taken to avoid neural damage.

Any resistance to injection must be assumed to indicate incorrect needle position, which requires adjustment, guided by the PNS, so that the needle is still in close proximity to the nerve but the subsequent injection is of low resistance.

Insulated versus uninsulated needles

There is no firm evidence as to whether the type of needle used is important in the success of the block or the risk of neural damage. A number of theories have been advanced to support both types of needle but there is no data to confirm any clinical benefit of insulated needles over uninsulated. From a practical perspective, uninsulated needles are widely available in a greater variety of length and diameter and are cheaper than insulated needles. For many peripheral nerve blocks uninsulated needles are entirely satisfactory with little loss of current along the length of the shaft. However, for deep nerves where the needle has to traverse a large muscle mass, e.g. the anterior approach to the sciatic nerve, the radial nerve (at the elbow) and the suprascapular nerve, insulated needles are recommended because they avoid localised direct stimulation of the muscles through which the needle passes. This direct stimulation can cause confusion about nerve location and uninsulated needles require up to twice the stimulus strength that insulated needles require.

The 'immobile needle'

This was first described by Winnie (1969) and uses a short (10–20 cm) extension tube to isolate the needle from movements of the syringe when performing peripheral nerve blockade. During aspiration, injection and syringe exchange, the needle can be held in a constant position, minimising the risks of nerve trauma and needle misplacement. It also allows the operator to use both hands to perform the technique and an assistant to make the injections.

Complications of regional anaesthesia

Introduction

Complications of peripheral neural blockade are uncommon provided that reasonable care is exercised in assessing the patient so that unsuitable patients are excluded and patient management is appropriate both during and after surgery. Complications range from the trivial to the life threatening and may be related to the block technique, the local anaesthetic used or the selection and management of the patient. Some complications are common to all blocks whilst others are specific to a particular technique. Specific side effects or complications are described in Section 3 under the individual techniques. No regional anaesthetic technique should be performed without the ability to monitor the patient, treat complications of the regional technique and administer general anaesthesia if necessary.

Complications of regional anaesthesia

For details of complications of regional anaesthesia see table provided below.

Technique	Patient	Drug
Neural damage	Pre-existing neural pathology	Intravascular injection
Haematoma	Inappropriate sedation	Drug overdose
Pneumothorax	Vasovagal faint	Anaphylactoid reaction
Widespread block	Faulty positioning	Excess vasoconstriction
Tourniquet pressure	Poor protection of affected area	'Wrong' solution
Compartment syndrome		
Methaemo-globinaemia		
Infection		

Complications of the technique

Neurological damage

Nerve damage is often cited as a reason to avoid practising regional anaesthesia, despite the very low incidence of neurological damage directly attributable to needle damage or other causes. The total number of regional anaesthetic blocks performed annually is unknown and the number of cases of nerve damage from both central and peripheral blocks is extremely small. It is impossible to determine the incidence of serious nerve damage, although several recent, very large studies have confirmed that permanent, serious morbidity is very rare. The great majority of post-operative neurological sequelae is temporary and typically manifests as sensory dysaesthesiae within the distribution of the affected nerve root(s) or the territory of a peripheral nerve. Recovery within a matter of days to a few weeks is the norm, although in a very small number of cases the damage is extensive and permanent. Neurological damage in patients undergoing general anaesthesia alone has been reported due to faulty positioning of the patient, surgical retraction and other unrelated causes. The femoral, ulnar, peroneal, lateral cutaneous nerve of thigh and the brachial plexus are at risk of compression due to over extension or flexion, and inadequate padding during prolonged surgery.

The most common injury is neuropraxia, where the nerve remains anatomically intact but individual nerve axons or bundles are functionally disrupted. Direct laceration by the needle tip is probably the most frequent cause of nerve damage, although the needle can damage the radicular arteries which accompany the nerves, causing ischaemic damage or compression by a localised haematoma. Other important and avoidable causes are firstly compression by hydraulic pressure within a rigid compartment, for example the ulnar nerve in the sulcus of the medial epicondyle of the humerus, and secondly over extension or flexion of limbs or the lumbar spine for prolonged periods.

Neurological damage from all causes can be minimised, if not entirely eliminated by close attention to the factors listed in Figure 1.15.

Haematoma formation

Within the spinal canal there is a rich plexus of epidural veins, which are prone to damage by spinal and epidural needles or catheters.

Figure 1.15
A strategy for minimising nerve damage from regional anaesthesia

- Sound anatomical knowledge
- Proper supervision and training
- Regular practice of the chosen technique
- Familiarity with the equipment
- Heightened awareness of potential difficulties
- Careful patient assessment and selection
- Attention to detail during surgical and anaesthetic management
- Gentleness, subtlety and care with the technique

In patients who have a fully functional clotting system, a damaged vein does not constitute a problem in terms of haematoma formation, but patients who have a clinical coagulopathy or who are receiving full anticoagulation may be exposed to an unacceptable risk of a haematoma. An epidural haematoma is a medical emergency because unless it is diagnosed early, preferably using magnetic resonance imaging (MRI), and surgically decompressed quickly (within a few hours of symptoms appearing) it will cause permanent neurological damage to the spinal cord. See p 12 for further advice regarding thrombo-prophylaxis and regional anaesthesia.

Many peripheral nerves run in close proximity to major vessels and inadvertent vascular puncture is a constant risk. In addition to the toxic effects of intravascular injection, extravasation and haematoma formation may distort local anatomical landmarks thus adding to the difficulty of nerve location and complicating the surgical approach. Other factors include increased patient discomfort, neural compression and subsequent neurological sequelae. If the patient has disordered clotting, the risks of such a complication must be weighed against the advantages and might preclude the use of some blocks where the risk of intravascular needle placement is high, for example axillary or subclavian brachial plexus, median nerve at the elbow, retrobulbar blocks.

Pneumothorax

The supraclavicular approaches to the brachial plexus, intercostal nerve, interpleural and thoracic paravertebral blocks have the potential to produce a pneumothorax. The published

figures for the incidence following brachial plexus blocks vary according to the use of confirmatory X-rays (complicated by the arbitrary assessment of volume and therefore clinical importance) but may be up to 6%. The sudden onset of pleuritic pain, dyspnoea or a dry cough may be the first sign of a pneumothorax which must be confirmed by chest X-ray, although pneumothorax may not present clinically for up to 24 h after the technique was performed. If the volume is significant (over 20% of the hemithorax) or if general anaesthesia with nitrous oxide is required, the pneumothorax must be drained. Usually pneumothoraces will resolve with conservative management and careful observation.

Widespread block

Central neural blocks can produce excessive blockade, resulting in dramatic hypotension, respiratory failure and loss of consciousness. An inappropriate volume of intrathecal local anaesthetic may spread to rostrally and produce a high thoracic or even cervical level of blockade, especially if head down tilt is used with a hyperbaric solution. An epidural block may turn into an accidental spinal due to inadvertent dural puncture by the needle or catheter and a large volume of local anaesthetic, intended for epidural use, may instead produce a total spinal injection, requiring immediate resuscitation.

Peripheral blocks that are performed adjacent to the central neuraxis (such as brachial plexus and paravertebral blocks) have the potential to spread centrally, thus producing bilateral effects. This may occur because of epidural block in the case of paravertebral blocks or by spread beneath the deep cervical fascia in the case of interscalene brachial plexus blocks. Brachial plexus blockade may also cause stellate ganglion blockade, inducing Horner's syndrome and phrenic nerve blockade, which may result in dyspnoea.

Infection

Infection is a rare but important complication of regional anaesthesia and may arise due to a faulty aseptic technique, by tracking from the site of skin puncture along the needle track or the percutaneous catheter. All major regional anaesthesia blocks should be performed using the same standard of sterility as a surgical procedure to reduce the risk to an absolute minimum. Infection complicating a peripheral nerve block is very uncommon and rarely gives rise to more than a localised infection, which is treated by systemic antibiotic therapy and removal of any indwelling catheter. However, infection complicating an epidural or spinal technique is a medical emergency either in the form of an epidural abcess or as meningitis. An epidural abcess has a similar compressive effect to a haematoma, with the additional complication of acting as a septic focus and requires urgent MRI, aggressive antibiotic treatment and surgical decompression. Meningitis may complicate both an epidural and a spinal, with all the typical features of photophobia, pyrexia, backache and neck stiffness. In the majority of cases, a causative organism may not be identified but a diagnostic lumbar puncture, culture of cerebrospinal fluid (CSF) and the catheter tip of the epidural catheter (if still in situ) or the puncture wound are mandatory.

Complications of patient management

Pre-existing neural pathology

Patients with pre-existing nerve damage due to diabetes mellitus, multiple sclerosis or other neurological diseases, require special consideration (see p 9, contraindications). Any post-operative deterioration in their neurological status will undoubtedly be attributed to the nerve block by the patient or the surgeons and nurses caring for them, despite any good evidence for this. Chronic neurological conditions such as multiple sclerosis may temporarily relapse following surgery whether or not regional anaesthesia is used. There is no clear evidence associating regional anaesthesia with adverse changes in neurological status, unless there is a clear contraindication to the use of a particular technique. For instance, the use of an epidural in someone with symptomatic spinal stenosis would be unwise. If there is clear clinical benefit to be gained from using a regional technique, pre-existing nerve lesions should be carefully documented pre-operatively and the patient should be thoroughly informed of the risks and benefits of the technique, which should be performed by an experienced practitioner of regional anaesthesia.

Inappropriate sedation

The decision about whether to sedate or anaesthetise a patient as part of the peri-operative management must be addressed carefully during the pre-operative visit. Inappropriate sedation can be difficult to manage, as the patient may become unco-operative, restless and even aggressive. Respiratory failure can occur unexpectedly in the elderly and cardiac arrest may ensue. It may be preferable to either have the patient completely awake and co-operative or to use a light general anaesthetic which is much more controllable, if the patient is unable to tolerate being fully conscious.

Vasovagal syncope

This common complication of regional anaesthesia can have serious consequences if not handled quickly and correctly. It may be volunteered by patients as evidence of a previous 'allergy' to local anaesthetic drugs and therefore needs careful discussion with the patient. Vasovagal events may occur in people other than the patient (nurses or other observers) when the technique is being performed, thus presenting the anaesthetist with two patients, one of who is now unconscious!

Faulty patient positioning

The manner in which the patient is positioned after the establishment of the block is important for two main reasons. Firstly, the anaesthetised portion of the body needs protection from pressure, high temperature and other potentially damaging forces as the patient will be unable to protect that part of their body in the normal way. Similarly hyperextension or flexion of anaesthetised joints must be avoided to prevent neural or cutaneous damage. Secondly, if the conscious patient is to undergo surgery lasting more than 30 min then they must be made as comfortable as possible to avoid increasing discomfort and consequent fidgeting and non-co-operation.

Tourniquet pressure

Pneumatic or elastic tourniquets are frequently used for limb or digit surgery and are associated with a risk of peripheral nerve and muscle damage if applied for a prolonged length of time or with excessive pressure over a small surface area. Careful control of total tourniquet time, padding of the cuff (which must be of the correct size) and appropriate inflation pressure will minimise such complications. If used in conjunction with peripheral nerve blockade, the tourniquet may cause patient discomfort if it is inflated on an unblocked part of the limb for more than a few minutes. The use of elastic tourniquets around the base of digits particularly if combined with digital nerve blocks can cause damage to the digital nerves and should be discouraged.

Compartment syndrome

Increased pressure in the myofascial compartments of a traumatised limb, due to oedema or haematoma, can cause muscular and neural damages from prolonged ischaemia. Pain on passive movement of the affected limb, tense swelling and decreased peripheral pulses are the cardinal signs. Urgent fasciotomy and excision of damaged tissue to prevent permanent nerve damage may be required. Many trauma patients are denied the benefits of a nerve block because of concerns that the block will mask the pain and thus delay diagnosis. If a patient is to undergo surgery to a limb that will decompress the affected compartments then regional anaesthesia is not contraindicated and may well increase perfusion of the affected area. If there is concern about compartment syndrome occurring at a later stage then intra-compartmental pressure monitoring should be instituted as a more sensitive monitor than the onset of pain. Careful post-operative monitoring of circulation and skin colour plus 'break through pain' is still necessary and full consultation with surgical colleagues should enable proper analgesia to be established without unnecessary risk.

Drug-related complications

Local anaesthetic drugs have very powerful membrane stabilising properties and can cause serious systemic cardiac and neurological toxicities. Unfortunately, partly because of the way in which they are traditionally labelled by percentage rather than in mg/ml concentration, many users are unaware of the concept of a safe

dose (either in volume or drug mass) and inject potentially lethal doses. The quoted maximum doses or volumes given on the drug data sheets by manufacturers are a guide but they do not allow for differences in clinical use. A particular dose may be perfectly safe if injected into a relatively avascular area but may cause systemic toxicity if injected into a very vascular area, due to rapid absorption.

Lidocaine is extensively used for treating cardiac dysrhythmias by decreasing the rate of depolarisation, the duration of the action potential and the refractory period. Bupivacaine is approximately four times more cardiotoxic than lidocaine due to its greater affinity for myocardial sodium channels and stronger binding capacity. It is associated with difficult resuscitation of ventricular dysrhythmias following the administration of a toxic dose and a number of deaths have been recorded due to failed resuscitation, even after prolonged attempts. Ropivacaine is intermediate in its toxicity profile – about twice as toxic as lidocaine and in the event of cardiac toxicity occurring, the evidence from animal experiments is that resuscitation is more successful than with bupivacaine.

See the chapter on *Local anaesthetic pharmacology* for a detailed discussion of drug-related complications.

'Wrong solutions'

This complication is one of bad management. If the technique is correctly carried out and all solutions are checked properly, then only a clearly labelled syringe of local anaesthetic agent should be available for the regional block. Ideally, all syringes containing local anaesthetic and adjuvant drugs for regional anaesthesia should be separated both in time and space from all other anaesthetic drugs and syringes. The local anaesthetic syringes should be filled by the person performing the injection and checked with a colleague before administration.

Management of complications

Most complications can be prevented by attention to detail in assessing the patient, planning and performing the block and in monitoring the patient closely during and after the operation. Minor adverse effects (light

Figure 1.16
Management of major adverse effects of regional anaesthesia

Psychological

- Distress
  - Reassurance
  - Supplementary oxygen
- Vasovagal syncope with bradycardia/hypotension
  - Atropine 600 mcg or glycopyrrolate 300 mcg i.v.
  - i.v. fluids
  - Consider ephedrine 3 mg increments i.v.

Anaphylactoid reactions

- Supplementary oxygen
- i.v. colloid
- Consider i.v. steroids/antihistamines

Anaphylactic reaction

- Intubation, ventilation with oxygen
- i.v. colloid
- Adrenaline 0.5 ml of 1:1000 initial dose i.v.
- Steroids (hydrocortisone 100–300 mg i.v.)
- Antihistamine (chlorpheniramine 10–20 mg i.v.)

Central nervous toxicity

- Mild
  - Supplementary oxygen
  - Reassurance
- Severe
  - Intubation, ventilation with oxygen
  - Anticonvulsants (diazepam/thiopentone increments)
  - Circulatory support

Cardiovascular depression

- Mild
  - Supplementary oxygen
  - Elevate legs
  - i.v. crystalloid
- Severe
  - Bradycardia: atropine 600 mcg i.v.
  - Hypotension: ephedrine 3 mg increments i.v.
  - Cardiopulmonary resuscitation as indicated by the relevant international body (for example European Resuscitation Council)

headedness, circumoral tingling) need no special treatment beyond stopping the injection. First line management of minor complications should follow a protocol, for example administer supplementary oxygen, monitor cardiovascular function and maintain verbal contact with the patient. The major adverse effects of intra-vascular injection of local anaesthetic are a medical emergency and require prompt and effective treatment as outlined in Figure 1.16.

Pharmacology of local anaesthetic drugs

Introduction

Local anaesthetic (LA) drugs work by reversibly blocking Na^+ ion selective receptors in the cell membranes of electrically excitable tissue, such as the nervous system and cardiac muscle. Within the peripheral nervous system, this has the effect of preventing depolarisation and onward neural transmission of noxious stimuli to the central neuraxis. Within the central nervous system (CNS), transmission between the afferent primary neurone and the interneurones of the dorsal horn is blocked, so interrupting the onward transmission of the stimuli towards the brain via second order ascending neurones. LAs also stabilise other membranes (such as myocardial muscle cells) and some (such as lidocaine) have clinically useful anti-dysrhythmic activity.

Nerve cell membrane anatomy and physiology

The membrane consists of a phospholipid bilayer, strengthened by cholesterol molecules that increase the symmetry of the highly motile hydrophobic tails while the hydrophilic heads add rigidity to the layer (Figure 1.17a). The membrane is interspersed with ion selective channels made of polypeptide subunits (Figure 1.17b). Each ion selective channel consists of several subunits that deform in response to changes in the voltage across the membrane and thus functionally open or close the channel.

There is a *resting potential* across human nerve membrane of approximately $-70\,mV$,

Figure 1.17
(a) A schematic view of an axonal nerve membrane. (b) A schematic cross section of a Na^+ channel

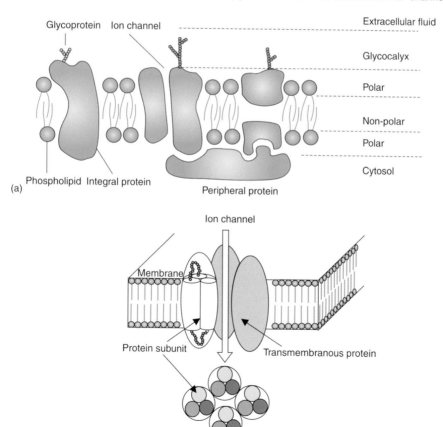

generated by the differential permeability of the membrane to Na$^+$ and K$^+$ ions. With the membrane at its resting potential of -70 mV, the Na$^+$ channels are closed and Na$^+$ is held outside the axon, whilst K$^+$ is largely an intracellular ion. The resting potential is maintained by the imbalance of the two ions across the membrane as K$^+$ is more permeable

Figure 1.18
(a) The Na$^+$/K$^+$ pump. (b) The phases of an action potential

than Na$^+$ and leaks out more readily than Na$^+$ can leak in. In addition, ATPase pumps within the nerve cell axon export three Na$^+$ ions from the axon in exchange for every two K$^+$ ions that move inwards (Figure 1.18a).

In response to a stimulus, neurotransmitters are released locally and generate a *slow potential*, which alters the protein structure of the axonal membrane, allowing Na$^+$ ions to enter the axoplasm and depolarise the membrane. If the stimulus is intense enough, the resting potential decreases by more than -20 mV (*the threshold potential*) and this stimulates an *action potential* of up to 110 mV (-70 to $+40$ mV). Na$^+$ ions rapidly cross the nerve membrane through the open ion channels and depolarise the membrane. A slower flow of K$^+$ ions in the reverse direction results in repolarisation. Ionic pumps restore the balance of ionic composition after repolarisation in the refractory phase (Figure 1.18b).

The action potential spontaneously replicates along the length of the axon at a *conduction velocity* that depends on the nerve fibre diameter and the degree of nerve fibre myelination. The velocity is much faster for large, myelinated Aα motor fibres than for small unmyelinated

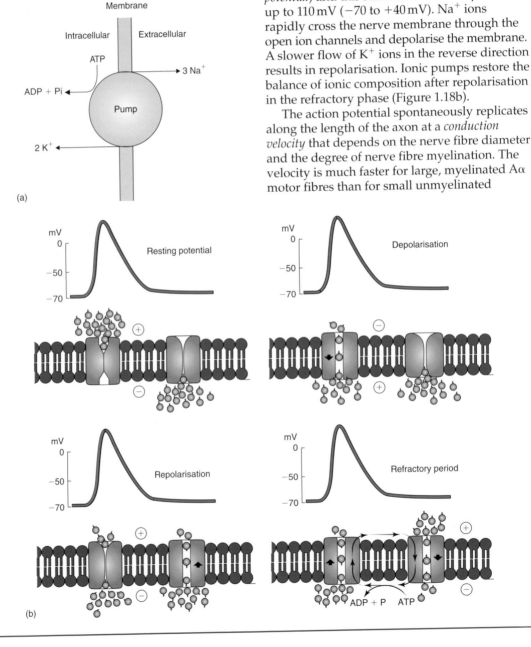

sensory c fibres. In unmyelinated fibres the action potential is a relatively slow continuous process but in myelinated fibres the Na^+ channels are concentrated at the nodes of Ranvier every 0.2–1.0 mm and the action potential spreads rapidly by jumping from node to node – Saltatory conduction.

Structure

All LA agents have an aromatic lipophilic tertiary amine head joined to an aminoalkyl hydrophilic tail by either an ester or an amide link (Figure 1.19). The head is derived from benzoic acid (esters) or alanine and the tail from ethyl alcohol, acetic acid or ringed piperidine. The link is 3–4 atoms long and confers structural orientation for receptor blockade as well as defining the method of metabolism. Changes to the basic structure, particularly to the tail, will alter the clinical properties of individual drugs by changing the geometric structure, potency, lipid and water solubility and toxicity. Mepivacaine, ropivacaine and bupivacaine all have the same head, amino link and piperidine ring tail but their increasing potency, duration of action and toxicity are a result of the increasing size of the side chain (methyl, propyl and butyl) on the piperidine ring (Figure 1.20).

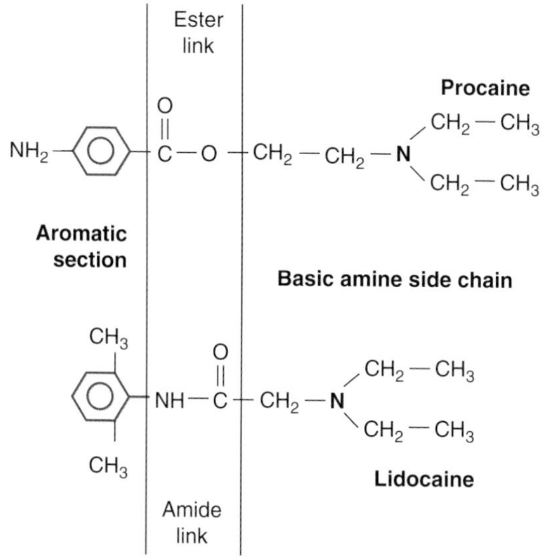

The ester linkage

The –COO– linkage is relatively unstable and the solutions have a short shelf life due to degradation of the link. The ester link is metabolised by plasma pseudocholinesterase, thus these drugs have a short clinical duration. Cocaine, procaine, chloroprocaine, benzocaine and amethocaine are all ester LAs.

The amide linkage

The –NHCO– bond is much stronger than the ester link. It produces more stable solutions, which are resistant to heat sterilisation and changes in pH. They also have a longer duration of action.

Some LAs have an asymmetric carbon atom linking the amide link to the tail (Figure 1.21). An asymmetric carbon atom has different atoms linked to each of its valency bonds and so the molecule can exist in more than one configuration (isomers). The molecule can exist in two mirror image forms – left handed (sinister (S)) or right handed (rectus (R)) (Figure 1.21). This is termed chirality. Each stereoisomer has differing properties including clinical effectiveness and toxicity. If the isomers rotate polarised light in opposite directions then they are optical stereoisomers and the direction of rotation varies for different drugs. The S form of bupivacaine and ropivacaine rotate light counterclockwise (−) and the R form rotates it clockwise (+) whereas for mepivacaine the reverse is true. Conventional drug manufacturing techniques produce a racemic mixture of both R and S forms that is optically neutral but new

Figure 1.19
Chemical structure of an ester (procaine) and an amide (lidocaine)

Figure 1.20
The variation of side chains for mepivacaine, ropivacaine and bupivacaine

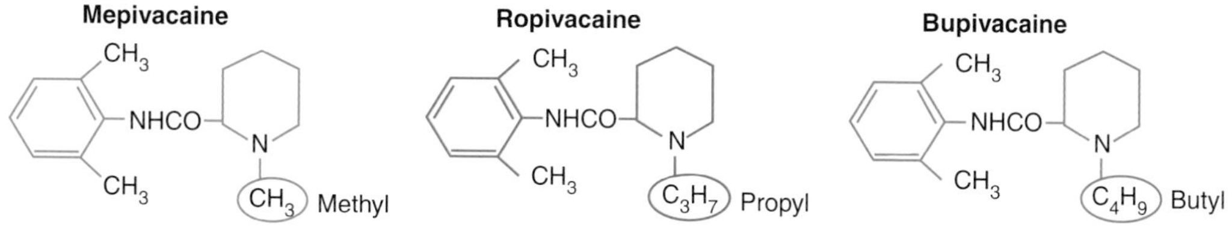

Figure 1.21
The optical isomers of ropivacaine

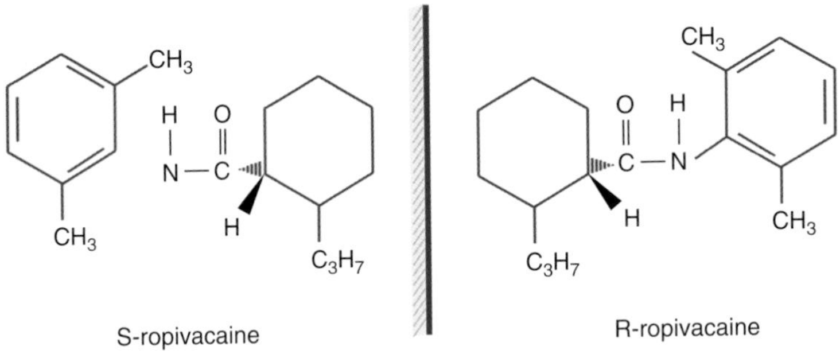

S-ropivacaine

R-ropivacaine

techniques of manufacture allow the production of just one isomer. As the R form of both bupivacaine and ropivacaine is more toxic and less clinically effective than the S form, both ropivacaine and S-bupivacaine are now available as pure S isomer formulations.

Mechanism of action

LA drugs are unionised, relatively water insoluble and unstable weak bases. They are therefore formulated as a crystalline salt – usually the hydrochloride to produce a water-soluble, stable drug. Within the ampoule, the LA is in acid solution with a high degree of ionisation that maintains solubility and stability. At physiological pH, the acid (ionised) and basic (non-ionised) components exist in equilibrium, the proportions of each component depending on the pKa of the drug and the ambient pH, as determined by the Henderson–Hasselbach equation (Figure 1.22).

Figure 1.22
The Henderson–Hasselbach equation for LA agents

$$pH = pKa + \frac{LA\ (base)}{LA\text{-}H^+\ (acid)}$$

The pKa for a given drug is constant and is the pH at which 50% of the drug is ionised and 50% unionised. The ratio of LA-base to LA-H$^+$ will therefore vary according to the ambient pH. Small changes in pH will have marked effects on the proportion of drug that is ionised which in turn influences both the transport across membranes and the clinical effect. The unionised LA-base is lipid soluble and diffuses

from the injection site through the epineurium, perineurium and across the nerve cell membrane into the axoplasm. Within the axoplasm, changes in ambient pH encourage ionisation, which produces the water-soluble cation (LA-H$^+$) by protonation of the highlighted amine nitrogen atom (Figure 1.23). This cation then binds electrostatically to the inner opening of the Na$^+$ channel, polarises the membrane and prevents onward transmission of the propagated action potential. As the unionised LA-base diffuses through the cell membrane, it produces a weak direct effect on the Na$^+$ channel, which accounts for about 10% of the total block. This is called *Phasic* or *Tonic* block and is caused by deformation of the polypeptide rods that make up the structure of the Na$^+$ channel. The channel does not need to be open for this affect to occur.

The pKa of lidocaine is 7.9, so (at pH 7.4) 24% is in the non-ionised state and 76% in the ionised state. The non-ionised drug is relatively lipophilic and passes passively down the concentration gradient through the membrane into the cell. The intracellular pH is about 7.1 and this shifts the balance of equilibrium within the axoplasm towards approximately 86% ionisation. The ionised drug, attracted by the negative charge of membrane protein then passes into the open ion channel, which remains open but is inactivated and further Na$^+$ flux is blocked.

Na$^+$ channels exist in three states – open, closed and inactive. LA cations bind preferentially to open channels and poorly to closed channels. When a cation binds to an open channel it becomes inactive and is no longer under voltage control. Thus, the quality of block is influenced by the state of the channels and the membrane polarity that controls them – the

Figure 1.23
Mechanism of action of LA action agents using lidocaine as an example

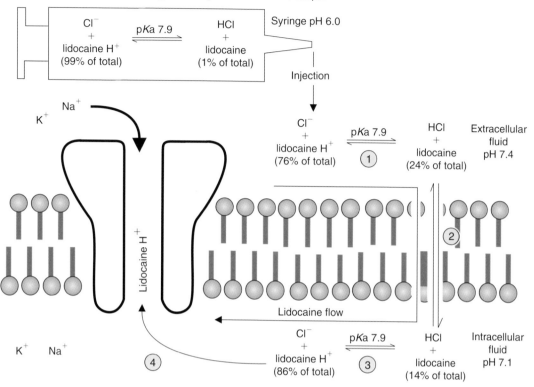

Figure 1.24
The Physicochemical and pharmacokinetic properties of important LA agents

	Molecular weight	pKa (25°C)	Partition coefficient	Protein binding (%)	Onset	Potency (relative to lido)	Duration
Esters							
Tetracaine	264	8.5	4.1	76	Slow	4	Long
Procaine	236	8.9	0.02	6	Slow	½	Short
Amides							
Bupivacaine	288	8.1	27.5	96	Medium	4	Long
Lidocaine	234	7.9	2.9	64	Rapid	1	Medium
Prilocaine	220	7.9	0.9	55	Rapid	1	Medium
Ropivacaine	274	8.1	6.1	95	Medium	4	Long

so-called *state-dependent block.* It follows that the more open channels there are, the more uptake of LA cations there will be and the more intense the resulting block. The higher the frequency of nerve stimulation, the more open channels there are and the more profound the block – this is the *frequency-dependent block* phenomenon and is important in understanding the basis of LA cardiac toxicity.

Factors influencing activity

Molecular weight, pKa, lipid solubility (expressed as a partition coefficient) and protein binding are the major physico-chemical properties of an LA drug, which govern its clinical activity. They also allow some prediction of comparative effects of different drugs (Figure 1.24).

Molecular weight

Molecular weight itself does not affect the pharmacological properties. However, increases in molecular weight tend to be indicative of increased side chain size and therefore increased potency and lipid solubility.

Lipid solubility

The higher the lipid solubility, the greater the penetration of the nerve membrane, so that higher lipid solubility results in greater potency. High lipid solubility also decreases the onset time and increases the duration of action of LA agents.

p*K*a

The lower the p*K*a, the lower the degree of ionisation for any given pH and so the more rapid the speed of onset of the block. Increasing the p*K*a increases the ionised proportion of the drug so that intracellularly a higher proportion is in the active state. However, this also means that less is in the non-ionised, diffusible state so the onset and offset of action are also slower. Figure 1.25 shows the effect of differences in pH and p*K*a on the proportion of ionised and non-ionised LA agents.

pH

The relationship between tissue pH and the p*K*a of the drug is crucial. If the difference between the two values is too great then the clinical effect of the drug will be inadequate. Either there will be excessive ionisation, which results in poor transmembrane transport but good Na^+ channel blocking or there will be a lack of ionisation, which results in good transport but poor Na^+ channel blocking. For example, acidosis at the site of injection will stimulate ionisation and reduce the amount of non-ionised drug available to cross the nerve membrane. Therefore, only a very small proportion of the initial dose is available for axoplasmic dissociation, reducing the final clinical potency. Conversely, if a drug has a low p*K*a, such as benzocaine (p*K*a = 3.5), then there will be little ionisation resulting in excellent transport across membranes but little clinical effect because of the lack of ionised cations. This is why benzocaine is only useful as a mucosal surface LA and only then in high

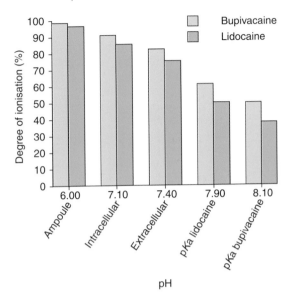

Figure 1.25
The effect of pH on the ionisation of LA agents

concentration (10–20%). Manipulation of the pH of the LA solution by addition of alkali, buffers, or carbonation may be used to alter the proportion of non-ionised drug.

Protein binding

The degree of protein binding reflects the ability of the drug to bind to membrane proteins; the greater the binding, the longer the duration of action. Increased binding to tissue protein correlates with an increase in the duration of action, and probably indicates a higher affinity for membrane proteins. Protein binding is also a predictor of LA toxicity because only the free (unbound) fraction of the drug is available for cardiac and neurological tissue binding. The higher the percentage of protein binding, the lower the free fraction is. The main binding sites within the plasma are alpha-1 acid glycoprotein, which has a high *affinity* but a low *capacity*, and albumin, which has a low *affinity* but a high *capacity* for LAs. Although plasma binding is important for intravascular levels of LA because it buffers changes in plasma concentration, the chemical bonds are weak and the protein readily releases the LA as concentration falls. Tissue binding is the more important factor when dealing with systemic toxicity because this determines how quickly LA will be absorbed from the site of injection into the vascular system.

LA toxicity

Clinical manifestations

All LAs produce central nervous and cardio-vascular effects as the free fraction (unbound) concentration in plasma rises above a threshold. The threshold concentration varies for each drug (the threshold for lidocaine is 4–5 mcg/ml) but individuals vary in their tolerance to LAs and there is no 'safe' plasma level. Acute clinical manifestations usually occur following direct intravascular injection because the drug mass is large enough to saturate the limited plasma binding capacity of albumin and alpha-1 glycoprotein. Intravascular injection is a risk with both central and peripheral nerve techniques because the epidural space contains a rich plexus of vessels and most large peripheral nerves accompany both veins and arteries in neurovascular bundles. Much of the published data on the toxic effects of intravascular injection relate to intravenous administration and the correlation between venous plasma levels and the observed symptoms. Intra-arterial injection is less common but extremely dangerous. In particular, blocks performed around the head and neck carry the attendant possibility of intra-arterial injection. Injection into the vertebral artery is a particular hazard of the interscalene approach to the brachial plexus when even a very small volume of LA will reach the cerebral circulation in high enough concentration to cause serious toxicity.

Serious toxicity is much less common following the systemic administration of a large therapeutic dose of LA because the binding capacity of the lungs and other tissue proteins ensures that most of the LA is not taken up by the blood stream. There have been a few deaths, however, following the use of lidocaine for liposuction, when exceptionally large doses have caused delayed systemic toxicity. Patients undergoing prolonged epidural or peripheral nerve catheter infusions may also report minor symptoms of toxicity.

The initial signs of toxicity are central nervous and cardiorespiratory excitation followed by generalised CNS and cardiovascular system (CVS) depression as the plasma levels progressively rise (Figure 1.26). The timescale and severity will vary according to a number of factors (Figure 1.27) but will tend to occur within a few seconds of the injection. The pattern of toxicity is broadly similar for all

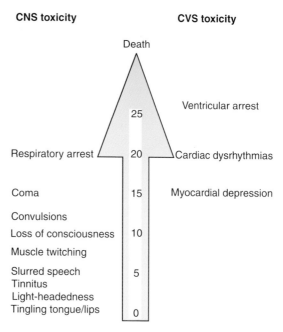

Figure 1.26
Signs of LA toxicity using lidocaine as an example

CNS toxicity		CVS toxicity
	Death	
	25	Ventricular arrest
Respiratory arrest	20	Cardiac dysrhythmias
Coma	15	Myocardial depression
Convulsions		
Loss of consciousness	10	
Muscle twitching		
Slurred speech	5	
Tinnitus		
Light-headedness		
Tingling tongue/lips	0	

Plasma lidocaine concentration (mcg/ml)

Figure 1.27
Factors influencing drug toxicity

- Molecular weight of the drug (related to its anaesthetic potency)
- Mass of drug injected
- Pharmacokinetic properties of the drug (affinity and binding capacity)
- Rate of rise of plasma levels
- Peak plasma level
- Total fraction of unbound drug in circulation

LA agents but variations exist in the relative severity of the cardiovascular and neurological effects. Bupivacaine has a narrower safety margin between CNS and cardiovascular toxicity than lidocaine and is particularly dangerous if cardiac effects do occur, as dissociation from the myocardium is slow, and successful resuscitation following cardiac arrest is unlikely unless prolonged cardiopulmonary resuscitation (CPR) is instituted.

CNS effects

The toxic CNS effects of LA agents are as follows:

- numbness and paraesthesiae of tongue, mouth and lips
- metallic taste
- light-headedness
- tinnitus
- slurred speech
- muscle twitching
- grand mal convulsions
- coma
- apnea

Apnea and convulsions result in hypoxia, hypercapnia and metabolic acidosis. The acidosis increases the proportion of ionised LA agent, which results in increased ion channel binding, so worsening the membrane stabilisation. Acidosis also effectively reduces the proportion of diffusible drug within the cells, and slows clearance.

CVS effects

Most LA agents (except cocaine) relax vascular smooth muscle causing vasodilatation. In addition, centrally administered drugs cause vasodilatation by sympathetic blockade. Direct cardiovascular toxicity occurs due to the membrane stabilising activity of the drugs on myocardial muscle, by blocking voltage-gated fast Na^+ channels. This reduces the maximum rate of rise of the cardiac action potential and reduces the duration of the action potential. Conduction of the action potential through the myocardium is slowed. Cardiac toxicity may result in any of the following effects:

- prolongation of PR interval
- supraventricular tachycardia
- decreased automaticity
- widening of QRS complex
- ventricular ectopic beats
- prolongation of ST interval
- T wave changes

Lidocaine is extensively used for treating cardiac dysrhythmias by decreasing the rate of depolarisation, the duration of the action potential and the refractory period. Bupivacaine is approximately four times more cardiotoxic than lidocaine due to its greater affinity for myocardial Na^+ channels and stronger binding capacity. It is associated with difficult resuscitation of ventricular dysrhythmias following the administration of a toxic dose and a number of deaths have been recorded due to failed resuscitation, even after prolonged attempts. Ropivacaine is intermediate in its toxicity profile – about twice as toxic as lidocaine and in the event of cardiac toxicity occurring, the evidence from animal experiments is that resuscitation is more successful than with bupivacaine.

Respiratory system

The respiratory effects of LA agents are due to a combination of peripheral neuronal blockade and systemic toxicity and the following effects may be seen.

- apnoea with systemic toxicity affecting the respiratory centre
- bronchodilatation secondary to relaxation of bronchial smooth muscle

Other effects

LA drugs have a weak neuromuscular blocking action. Amides block plasma cholinesterase. A direct anti-platelet effect (probably due to membrane stabilisation) reduces platelet aggregation and blood viscosity. These effects are of minor clinical significance.

Anaphylactoid reactions

Anaphylactoid reactions are very rare with amide LAs, and some of those reported have been due to preservatives (such as metabisulphite and methylparaben). Effects range from local erythema and swelling to systemic hypotension and bronchospasm. More commonly, the reactions are due to co-administration of adrenaline, intravascular injection or psychological effects (vasovagal episodes). Reactions are more common with esters and cross sensitivity may occur. The metabolism of procaine produces para-amino benzoic acid (PABA) which may be allergenic. Careful history taking will determine the likely cause of any previous adverse reaction and if necessary the patient should undergo a series of skin testing injections to confirm whether true allergy exists.

Factors affecting LA toxicity

CVS and CNS toxicity depend on the mass of drug reaching the systemic circulation. The

Figure 1.28
The maximum recommended doses (and their mg/kg equivalents) for various LA agents

	Adult dose (mg)		mg/kg equivalent	
	Plain	With adrenaline	Plain	With adrenaline
Ester				
Cocaine	100	*	1.6	*
Amide				
Bupivacaine	150	150	2	2
Lidocaine	200	500	3	7
Prilocaine (felypressin)	400	600 (felypressin)	6	8.5
Ropivacaine	250**	n/a	3.5	n/a

*Unnecessary and contraindicated.
**150 mg (32 mg/kg) for epidural Caesarean section.

transfer of drug (by diffusion) from the circulation to organs is determined by the Fick principle. The mass of drug reaching the circulation after peripheral administration is influenced by the following factors:

- mass of drug administered
- site of injection
- tissue protein binding and metabolism
- vascularity of the injection site

Dose

The volume and concentration of LA agents, considered individually, have little influence on systemic spread. Systemically the mass of drug rather than its administered concentration is more important. Figure 1.28 lists maximum recommended doses.

Absorption

Absorption from different sites is influenced by the blood flow to the tissue and the uptake of the drug into vascular compartment, which is a function of solubility. Absorption is in the order of magnitude:

Intercostal > epidural > plexus > peripheral > subcutaneous

Absorption is particularly high when agents are applied topically to mucosa (such as lidocaine spray in the oropharynx). A vasoconstrictor may be added to reduce absorption. Cocaine produces vasoconstriction in its own right and is used on the nasal mucosa to reduce vascularity prior to some ear, nose and throat (ENT) procedures.

Accidental intravenous injection bypasses the absorption process and subjects the patient to potentially toxic levels of drug. Intravenous regional anaesthesia (IVRA) involves the deliberate introduction of LA into the venous system of a limb isolated by tourniquet. The safety of this procedure is dependent on the drug becoming predominantly tissue bound by the time the tourniquet is released, which should not be less than 20 min. Further improvements in safety can be achieved by using relatively non-cardiotoxic drugs, typically prilocaine.

Distribution

Absorbed drug passes through the lungs where a large amount of the LA agent may become tissue bound and in some cases metabolised. However, this capacity is rapidly saturated following direct intravenous injection. After passing through the lungs LA drugs reach vessel rich tissues which have a high affinity. Some is distributed to muscle and fat, and later gradually released for subsequent metabolism.

Metabolism

Ester LAs are rapidly metabolised by plasma and liver cholinesterases (including pseudocholinesterase) and systemic toxicity is rarely a problem. Amide LAs are all tertiary amines (except prilocaine, which is a secondary amine) and are metabolised by the liver. They are dealkylated in the liver to secondary amines before further oxidative dealkylation and hydroxylation. Hepatic failure must be very severe before LA breakdown is compromised.

Lidocaine has a high extraction ratio and metabolism is therefore dependent on hepatic blood flow, which may be particularly relevant when intravenous lidocaine is used to stabilise ventricular myocardium in low cardiac output states.

Pregnancy

Fetal blood rapidly equilibrates with maternal blood levels of the free fraction of LA agent, but as there is less alpha-1 acid glycoprotein in fetal blood, the overall concentration will be higher. The pH of the fetal fluids is lower than maternal which increases the proportion of ionised LA agent. Metabolism is less well developed in the foetus but the drug rapidly passes back to the mother as maternal levels decline, therefore this does not present a problem. Neurobehavioural studies of neonates born following epidural anaesthesia show no clinical effects related to absorption of bupivacaine or ropivacaine.

Ester linked LAs

Tetracaine

Tetracaine (amethocaine) is used for topical anaesthesia. It is available as a 4% gel and is indicated for local anaesthesia of the skin before intravascular cannulation. It is effective within 45 min. The preparation should not be applied to inflamed or damaged skin or highly vascular tissues as it is rapidly absorbed through mucosal surfaces. More dilute solutions (0.5% and 1%) are available for topical anaesthesia of the conjunctiva. Tetracaine is potent and readily absorbed but in common with other ester LAs, it may cause hypersensitivity.

Benzocaine

Benzocaine is unusual in that the side chain is an ethyl group with no amine component and therefore remains unionised. Benzocaine has a low potency but it may cause methaemo-globinaemia. It is a component of some throat lozenges, and may be applied directly to painful skin ulcers.

Cocaine

Cocaine is a naturally occurring ester derived from benzoic acid, and extracted from the leaves of *Erythroxylum coca*. It is available in solution and pastes ranging from 1% to 10% concentrations. It is mainly used for topical anaesthesia and to reduce bleeding during nasal surgery. Cocaine is rapidly taken up into mucous membranes to provide anaesthesia and intense vasoconstriction. This vasoconstriction limits systemic absorption resulting in a bioavailability by this route of 0.5%. It is well known as a drug of abuse with high addictive potential, and in this role is taken by chewing, inhaling nasally, smoking or intravenously. It causes marked sympathomimetic activity and dysrhythmias are a serious risk. Systemic injection must be avoided. Systemically absorbed cocaine has a volume of distribution of 2 l/kg with 98% being protein bound. It is eliminated by plasma and liver esterases, having a clearance of 35 ml/kg/min and a half-life of 45 min.

Cocaine (pKa = 8.7) shares the same mechanism of action as the other LA agents and also inhibits catecholamine neuronal uptake. Synaptic levels of dopamine and noradrenaline increase, resulting in central stimulation, euphoria and vasoconstriction. Cocaine initially blocks the inhibitory pathways resulting in euphoria, hyperthermia, altered vision and hearing, nausea and eventually convulsions. The central stimulation increases respiratory rate and volume. A rise in sympathetic tone leads to tachycardia and hypertension; the latter is exacerbated by peripherally mediated vasoconstriction. Higher levels of cocaine also block the excitatory pathways resulting in central nervous depression leading to sedation, unconsciousness and respiratory depression. Cocaine causes mydriasis and raised intra-ocular pressure and is no longer used for local anaesthesia of the eye. High doses depress the myocardium. The general excitation also increases metabolic rate, which contributes to the hyperthermia and raises oxygen consumption and carbon dioxide production. The recommended maximum dose is 1.5 mg/kg. Cocaine should be avoided in porphyria.

Amides

Bupivacaine

Bupivacaine is a long-acting LA agent with a slow onset of action. Blockade of a large peripheral nerve, such as the sciatic nerve, may take 60 min depending on the approach but may last up to 48 h. Intrathecal injection, by contrast, produces an acceptable block within a few minutes. Bupivacaine has been associated with a number of deaths from cardiac toxicity where resuscitation was prolonged and difficult. These cases stimulated the search for safer long-acting amide LAs and resulted in the development of the pure S isomers (alternatively named levo) of ropivacaine and bupivacaine. The S forms have a lower cardiac and neurological toxicity as well as a slightly more potent clinical effect than the R form and the racemic mixture. Recommendations to minimise systemic toxicity specific to bupivacaine include:

- avoid bupivacaine for IVRA
- avoid 0.75% bupivacaine in obstetric practice
- limit dose to 2 mg/kg

Bupivacaine is predominantly metabolised by N-dealkylation to pipecolyloxylidine. N-desbutylbupivacaine and hydroxybupivacaine are also produced. The metabolites are excreted in the urine.

Lidocaine (lignocaine)

Lidocaine is primarily an LA agent but is also a Class IB anti-dysrhythmic.

Lidocaine has a relatively rapid onset of action and intermediate duration. Combination with a longer-acting agent, such as bupivacaine, may produce an intermediate onset time and duration compared to each of the component agents. The cardiotoxic potential of lidocaine at equivalent levels of central nervous toxicity is about 1/9 that of bupivacaine.

Lidocaine is metabolised in the liver by micro-somal oxidases and amidases. N-dealkylation followed by hydrolysis produces ethylglycine, xylidide and other derivatives that are excreted in the urine.

Prilocaine

Prilocaine is similar to lidocaine in terms of pharmacological activity. It has the same pKa (7.9) but is less lipid soluble. Speed of onset and duration are similar. It is less toxic than lidocaine, due to high tissue fixation, and rapid metabolism of systemically absorbed drug. Prilocaine is the drug of choice for IVRA.

Prilocaine is metabolised in the liver, lungs and kidney to O-toluidine, and then hydroxytoluidine, leaving less than 1% unchanged. If a large quantity of prilocaine is used, more than 10 mg/kg, sufficient O-toluidine is produced to cause *methaemoglobinaemia* from the oxidation of the ferrous ion (Fe^{2+}) of the haem in haemoglobin to ferric (Fe^{3+}). If more than 10% of the haemoglobin is converted to methaemoglobin cyanosis will be observed and pulse oximeter readings dip towards 85%, despite normal oxygen saturation. Methaemoglobinaemia is not usually clinically detrimental but if the patient is compromised, slow intravenous injection of methylene blue (1–2 mg/kg) may be used as a treatment. Excess methylene blue (>7 mg/kg) may also cause methaemoglobinaemia, and as the dye has a distinctive spectral absorption it also affects pulse oximeter accuracy. Children (especially infants) are more susceptible to methaemoglobinaemia because they have under developed metabolic processes and fetal haemoglobin is more easily oxidised. Methaemoglobinaemia also occurs occasionally after application of eutectic mixture of local anaesthetic (EMLA) cream, which contains prilocaine.

Ropivacaine

Ropivacaine is closely related to bupivacaine in terms of pharmacological activity as both drugs are pipecoloxylidides. Ropivacaine was the first LA agent produced as a single enantiomer (bupivacaine is a racemic mixture) which has an enantiometric purity of 99.5% for S-ropivacaine. As ropivacaine is less lipid soluble than bupivacaine and less readily penetrates the neuronal myelin sheaths, C fibres are blocked more readily than A fibres. At high concentrations, the blocking effect is similar for both drugs but at lower concentrations ropivacaine preferentially blocks C fibres compared to A fibres. Ropivacaine has a potential advantage that motor function can be spared (or show earlier recovery) whilst still achieving sensory blockade, if a suitable concentration of drug is used. Complete motor and sensory blockade can still be achieved if desired. In summary, ropivacaine provides sensory blockade similar to that of bupivacaine but motor blockade is slower in onset, less pronounced and shorter in duration. Ropivacaine is half as cardiotoxic as racemic bupivacaine and there is some evidence that it may be slightly less toxic than S-bupivacaine.

EMLA

EMLA is a mixture of 2.5% prilocaine and 2.5% lidocaine used for topical anaesthesia of undamaged skin before intravascular cannulation and minor, very superficial dermal surgery. A eutectic mixture is one in which the constituents are in such proportions that the freezing (or melting) point is as low as possible, with the constituents freezing (or melting) simultaneously. The preparation is therefore unusual, as the LAs are not in aqueous solution, and both agents are in their pure form rather than the hydrochloride preparations used in the solutions. In theory, this means that both drugs are in the non-ionised state in EMLA and that ionisation will occur after absorption has occurred. The commercial preparation (EMLA cream 5%) contains carboxypolymethylene and sodium hydroxide resulting in an oil–water emulsion.

Additives

Glucose

Standard solutions of LA agents are slightly hypobaric at body temperature and pH and therefore tend to move upwards in the cerebrospinal fluid away from the gravitational pull. Dextrose (glucose) is added to bupivacaine to increase the density of the solution. The specific gravity of hyperbaric (or 'heavy') bupivacaine is 1.026 at 20°C. The specific gravity of cerebrospinal fluid is 1.005 at 37°C, so the injected bupivacaine solution will sink due to gravity. This helps to control the distribution of the LA using knowledge of the spinal curves and by manipulating the position of the patient.

Note: the specific gravity of a substance or solution is the density of that solution relative to the maximum density of water, which occurs at a temperature of 4°C.

Vasoconstrictors

Epinephrine (adrenaline)

Epinephrine is added to LA solutions to reduce vascularity of the area by direct vasoconstriction and in turn reduce the systemic uptake of the drug. This has the following effects:

- increased duration of nerve blockade
- greater margin of safety for systemic toxicity
- reduced surgical bleeding

Care must be taken to avoid the systemic effects of epinephrine due to systemic uptake. For example, combination with halothane anaesthesia may result in cardiac dysrhythmias, especially ventricular excitation and fibrillation. Epinephrine-containing solutions should not be injected in the proximity of end-arteries, such as the penile, ophthalmic (central artery of the retina), or digital arteries as there is no collateral circulation to supplement the supply if vasoconstriction is severe. To minimise the risk of serious systemic actions consider the following:

- avoid hypoxia and hypercarbia
- use dilute solutions less than 1:200,000
- limit of 200 mcg per 10 min
- limit of 300 mcg per hour

The concentration of epinephrine in most commercially available solutions of LA is 1:200,000 (5 mcg/ml). An injection of 40 ml (during a brachial plexus block for example) will therefore contain 200 mcg and should be considered as a maximum dose for a single injection. An intravascular injection of only 2–3 ml of a LA solution containing epinephrine will cause the patient to experience tachycardia, hypertension, palpitations and a feeling of apprehension.

A solution containing epinephrine is more acid than the equivalent plain solution and may contain sodium chloride to maintain isotonicity. It may also contain preservatives, such as sodium metabisulphite or methylparahydroxybenzoate.

Felypressin

Felypressin is an octapeptide derived from vasopressin (ADH). In common with vasopressin, felypressin is a powerful direct-acting vasopressor, but it is safe to use with halothane and has no antidiuretic or oxytocic activity. It may, however, cause coronary vasoconstriction.

Hyaluronidase

Hyaluronidase, supplied as a white powder, is used to facilitate the spread through connective tissues following subcutaneous or intra-muscular injection. In addition to promoting the spread of LAs and other injections, it is also used to promote reabsorption of fluids and

Figure 1.29
Analgesia adjuvants to LAs, used for receptor-mediated analgesic effect

Drug	Receptor	Site
Opioids	μ/κ	Central and peripheral
Clonidine	α_2-adrenergic	Central and peripheral
Ketamine	NMDA	Central
Neostigmine	Cholinergic	Central and peripheral

Figure 1.30
Structures of common LA drugs

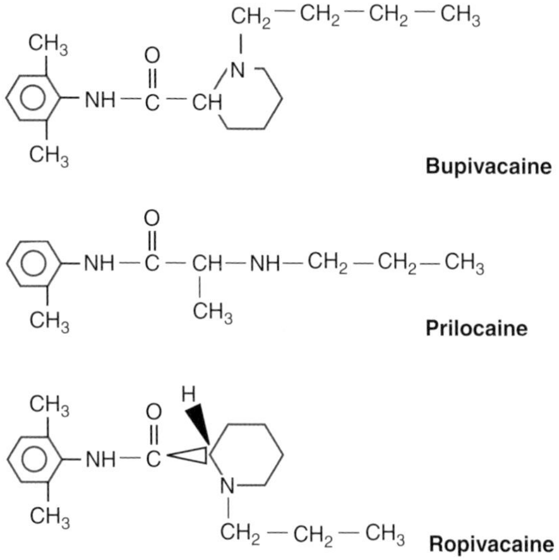

Bupivacaine

Prilocaine

Ropivacaine

blood from extravascular tissues. Its effect is dependent on the temporary depolymerisation of hyaluronic acid. Hyaluronidase is stable in solution for 24 h at room temperature.

pH manipulation

Carbonation of LA agents may increase the speed of onset and the depth of the block. The carbon dioxide diffuses out of the injected LA and increases tissue pH. This results in a higher proportion of non-ionised drug, which diffuses into the neurone more rapidly. Preparation and storage is awkward and the preparations are not widely available. Alkalisation of solutions by addition of bicarbonate is comparable.

Additives with analgesic activity

A number of adjuvant drugs are now used to provide a synergistic effect on pain perception by interaction with specific receptors in the afferent pathways (Figure 1.29).

Specific pharmacology

Units (unless stated otherwise) are as follows:

- volume of distribution at steady state (Vd)   l/kg
- clearance (Cl)   ml/kg/min
- terminal half-life ($t_{1/2}$)   hours

Bupivacaine hydrochloride

Structure amide LA agent, pipecoloxylidide (Figure 1.30).

Presentation clear, colourless, aqueous solutions include:

- plain solutions (0.25%, 0.5%, 0.75%)
- solutions with 1:200,000 (5 mcg/ml) adrenaline (0.25%, 0.5%)
- 'heavy' 0.5% with 80 mg/ml dextrose (specific gravity 1.026) for spinal anaesthesia

Recommended maximum dose 2 mg/kg (150 mg plus up to 50 mg 2 hourly subsequently).
Pharmacokinetics

Molecular weight	pKa	Partition coefficient	Protein binding	Vd	Cl	$t_{1/2}$
288	8.1	27.5	95%	1	7	30

Clinical intermediate speed of onset, long action, four times as potent as lidocaine; propensity to cardiotoxicity.
Elimination 5% excreted as pipecoloxylidine after dealkylation in the liver, 16% excreted unchanged in urine.

s-bupivacaine hydrochloride (levobupivacaine)

Structure amide LA agent, pipecoloxylidide.
Presentation clear, colourless, aqueous solutions of plain solutions (0.25%, 0.5%, 0.75%).
Recommended maximum dose 2 mg/kg (maximum of 400 mg in 24 h).

Pharmacokinetics

Molecular weight	pKa	Partition coefficient	Protein binding	Vd	Cl	t$_{1/2}$
288	8.1	27.5	>97%	1	9	80

Clinical intermediate speed of onset, long action, four times as potent as lidocaine; less cardiotoxic and neurotoxic than racemic bupivacaine.
Elimination 100% metabolism to 3-hydroxy-levobupivacaine via CYP3A4 and CYP1A2 pathways in liver; 71% eliminated via urine and 24% in faeces within 48 h.

Lidocaine hydrochloride

Structure amide LA agent, derivative of diethylaminoacetic acid.
Preparation clear, aqueous solutions include:

- plain solutions (0.5%, 1%, 2%)
- solutions with 1:200,000 (5 mcg/ml) adrenaline (0.5%, 1%, 2%)
- gel (2%) with and without chlorhexidine for urethral instillation
- solutions for surface application to pharynx, larynx and trachea (4%) (coloured pink)
- spray for anaesthesia of the oral cavity and upper respiratory tract (10%)

Dose topical, infiltration, nerve blocks, epidural and spinal; 0.5–10% available; 100 mg bolus then 1–4 mg/min for ventricular dysrhythmias.
Recommended maximum dose 200 mg (3 mg/kg); with adrenaline 500 mg (7 mg/kg)
Pharmacokinetics

Molecular weight	pKa	Partition coefficient	Protein binding	Vd	Cl	t$_{1/2}$
234	7.9	2.9	64%	1	9	100

Clinical rapid speed of onset, intermediate action; Class IB anti-dysrhythmic.
Elimination 70% by dealkylation in liver, less than 10% excreted unchanged in urine.

Prilocaine hydrochloride

Structure amide LA agent, secondary amine derived from toluidine.
Preparation clear, colourless, aqueous solutions include:

- plain solutions (0.5%, 1%, 2%, 4%)
- solutions with 0.03 unit/ml felypressin (3%)

Recommended maximum dose 400 mg (= 6 mg/kg); with felypressin 600 mg (= 8.5 mg/kg)
Pharmacokinetics

Molecular weight	pKa	Partition coefficient	Protein binding	Vd	Cl	t$_{1/2}$
220	7.9	0.9	55%	3.7	40	261

Clinical rapid speed of onset, intermediate duration of action between lidocaine and bupivacaine, potency similar to lidocaine; may result in methaemoglobinaemia.
Elimination rapidly metabolised to *O*-toluidine by liver, less than 1% excreted unchanged.

Ropivacaine hydrochloride

Structure amide LA agent, pipecoloxylidide (Figure 1.30).
Presentation clear, colourless, aqueous solutions of *s*-ropivacaine enantiomer include:

- plain solutions in 10 and 20 ml ampoules (2, 7.5, 10 mg/ml)
- plain solution in 100 and 200 ml bags (2 mg/ml) for epidural infusion

Recommended maximum dose 250 mg (150 mg for Caesarean section under epidural); cumulative dose of 675 mg over 24 h according to data so far.
Pharmacokinetics

Molecular weight	pKa	Partition coefficient	Protein binding	Vd	Cl	t$_{1/2}$
274	8.1	6.1	94%	0.8	10	110

Clinical intermediate onset, long duration of action between lidocaine and bupivacaine, potency similar to lidocaine; greater separation of sensory and motor blockade, and lower cardiotoxicity than bupivacaine may be advantages.
Elimination aromatic hydroxylation to 3- (and 4-) hydroxy-ropivacaine, and *N*-dealkylation; 86% (mostly conjugated) excreted in the urine, of which 1% is unchanged; 3- and 4-hydroxy-bupivacaine have reduced LA activity.
Contraindication IVRA, obstetric paracervical block; not yet recommended in children under 12 years of age.

Introduction

This section is divided into four anatomical regions – the lower extremity, the trunk, the upper extremity and the head and neck (including ophthalmic local blocks). There is a common layout describing the relevant anatomy of the nerve supply and important topographical landmarks, the indications for the nerve block techniques and appropriate surgical procedures. Finally the peripheral nerve blocks for each region are described in detail, starting with the proximal plexuses or nerve trunks and working distally to the smaller nerve trunks and terminal nerves.

1. Certain practical details will be common to most, if not all, regional blocks where short bevelled needles are used to perform the technique. Patient management, safe sedation practice, basic physiological monitoring and the requirements for block performance are described in Section 1.
2. The Peripheral Nerve Stimulator is an important instrument in successful peripheral nerve blocks and its use is described in detail in Section 1.
3. Conscious patients require local anaesthetic infiltration of the skin and subcutaneous tissues at the needle insertion point to ensure that the regional block technique is well tolerated. Lidocaine 1% injected through a 25G hypodermic needle is almost painless for the majority of patients if done slowly and gently. Some stinging can be expected and if tissue distension is rapid this can be painful for the patient until the lidocaine works. Skin infiltration done slowly and carefully should be almost painless but anxious or needle-phobic patients can be offered a topical local anaesthetic cream over the site of injection.

These important points are assumed to apply to all of the techniques described in this section. They will not be referred to under individual techniques unless there are specific reasons for doing so.

The lower extremity

Introduction

The lumbar and sacral segmental nerve roots of the spinal cord provide the nerve supply to the lower extremity by forming two plexuses (lumbar and sacral), which in turn produce five major terminal nerves. The femoral nerve, obturator nerve and lateral cutaneous nerve of thigh (LCNT) are the terminal nerves of the lumbar plexus to the lower extremity and the sciatic plexus produces the sciatic nerve and the posterior cutaneous nerve of thigh.

The five major terminal nerves to the lower limb can be blocked at a number of sites from the level of the lumbar and sacral plexuses down to the malleoli. The area of anaesthesia can be extended or restricted according to the site of surgery and the degree of motor and sensory block required by performing the peripheral nerve blocks at the most appropriate level.

The upper leg and hip joint
Anatomy
Lumbar plexus

The lumbar plexus is formed from the anterior divisions of L1–4 (Figure 2.1) within the substance of the psoas major muscle, in front

Figure 2.1
The lumbar plexus

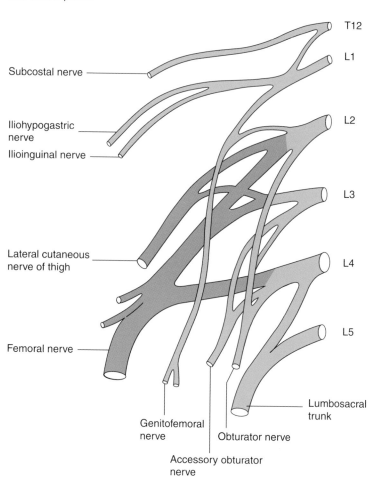

Subcostal nerve

Iliohypogastric nerve

Ilioinguinal nerve

Lateral cutaneous nerve of thigh

Femoral nerve

Genitofemoral nerve

Accessory obturator nerve

Obturator nerve

Lumbosacral trunk

T12

L1

L2

L3

L4

L5

of the transverse processes of the lumbar vertebrae. The lumbar plexus forms six terminal nerves; three proximal ones – iliohypogastric, ilioinguinal (T12–L1) and genitofemoral (L1, 2), supply motor and sensory branches to the lower abdomen, external genitalia and the inner aspect of the skin of the thigh (see p 72).

The three distal nerves of the plexus, the femoral nerve (L2, 3, 4), the LCNT (L2, 3) and the obturator nerve (L2, 3, 4) provide sensory and motor innervation to the anterior aspects of the upper leg with a sensory branch of the femoral nerve descending as far distally as the medial malleolus as the saphenous nerve.

Femoral nerve

The femoral nerve is the largest branch of the plexus. It emerges from the distal lateral border of the psoas muscle, passing beneath the inguinal ligament immediately lateral to the femoral vessels. Distal to the inguinal ligament, the nerve is deep to the fascia lata and is encased within the layers of the ilio-pectineal fascia. It divides into anterior and posterior divisions just distal to the inguinal ligament. The anterior division supplies the sartorius muscle and skin of the anterior and medial aspects of the thigh, including the knee. The posterior division supplies motor fibres to the quadriceps femoris, vastus medialis and lateralis and sensory fibres to the knee joint. It continues distal to the knee joint as the saphenous nerve.

Obturator nerve

The obturator nerve leaves the psoas muscle on the postero-medial side and passes through the obturator foramen of the pelvis into the medial part of the upper leg. It divides into a posterior and anterior branch, separated by the adductor brevis muscle. Both branches supply motor nerves to the adductor muscles and sensory fibres, which have a variable sensory distribution to the skin on the medial aspect of the thigh and the capsule of the knee joint. The anterior branch supplies sensory fibres to the hip and the medial aspect of the thigh and the posterior branch supplies the knee.

LCNT

The LCNT emerges from the midpoint of the lateral border of the psoas muscle and is the most proximal of the three main nerves to the lower limb. It passes laterally and distally along the ilium, lying on the surface of the iliacus muscle, until it passes deep to the inguinal ligament about 1 cm medial to the anterior superior iliac spine (ASIS). It provides sensory innervation to a variable area of skin on the antero-lateral aspect of the thigh from the level of the greater trochanter down to the level of the knee, although the innervated area may be much smaller than this (Figure 2.2).

Applied anatomy

There is an anatomical continuity from the epidural space, where the segmental nerve roots emerge, through the paravertebral space and the psoas muscle compartment to the distal border of the psoas where the femoral nerve is enveloped in its sheath. The lumbar plexus and

Figure 2.2
Cutaneous innervation of LCNT

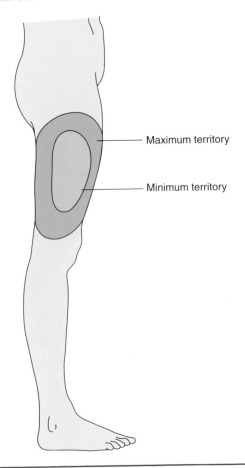

Maximum territory

Minimum territory

its terminal nerves can therefore be blocked either proximally or distally. The lumbar paravertebral approach blocks the nerve roots before they enter the psoas muscle and the psoas compartment or sheath technique blocks the components of the plexus within the psoas muscle. The plexus can also be approached by a distal technique known as the inguinal paravascular or '3 in 1' block. This latter approach relies on a retrograde spread of local anaesthetic within the femoral nerve sheath and blocks all three nerves of the plexus less consistently than the proximal approaches. In children and young adults, the iliacus block has been used with some success but is less reliable in adults.

Sacral plexus

The sacral plexus (Figure 2.3) is formed from the lumbosacral trunk (the ventral rami of L4–5 and the ventral rami of S1, 2, 3). The plexus lies on the piriformis muscle over the anterior surface of the sacrum and gives rise to several pelvic and gluteal branches within the pelvis but only two terminal nerves to the lower limb. The sciatic nerve and the posterior cutaneous nerve of thigh both leave the pelvis through the

Figure 2.3
The sacral plexus

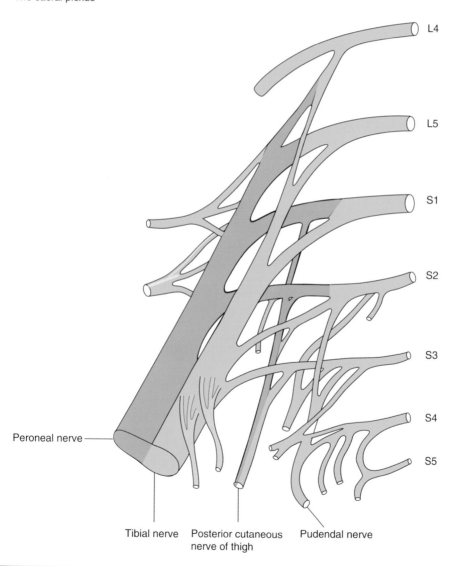

L4
L5
S1
S2
S3
S4
S5

Peroneal nerve

Tibial nerve   Posterior cutaneous   Pudendal nerve
nerve of thigh

greater sciatic foramen and are in close proximity as they descend down the back of the thigh. The sciatic nerve is the largest and longest peripheral nerve and supplies motor and sensory innervation to the posterior aspect of the upper and lower leg, terminating in the nerves to the foot at the level of the malleolii. The posterior cutaneous nerve of thigh is closely applied to the sciatic nerve as far as the midpoint of the thigh and then becomes subcutaneous.

Sciatic nerve

The sciatic nerve (L4, 5, S1, 2, 3) is the largest nerve in the body – up to 2.5 cm wide as it exits the pelvis. It has two component nerves (peroneal and tibial nerves), which are usually joined together when the sciatic nerve emerges from the sciatic foramen. They divide into separate nerves at a variable level, anywhere from the sciatic foramen to the popliteal fossa. In the thigh, the sciatic nerve supplies articular branches to the hip joint and motor branches to the hamstring muscles. The terminal nerves supply most of the cutaneous innervation below the knee (Figure 2.4).

Posterior cutaneous nerve of the thigh

The posterior cutaneous nerve of the thigh (S1, 2, 3) runs postero-medial to the sciatic nerve deep to fascia lata and innervates the posterior aspect of the thigh. At the apex of the popliteal fossa it pierces the deep fascia and continues into the proximal part of the calf, supplying the overlying skin and subcutaneous tissue of the upper part of the calf.

Applied anatomy

The sacral plexus lies immediately anterior to the sacrum and is not amenable to direct plexus blockade. In theory, it can be approached via the trans-sacral foraminae but this requires four separate injections, each of which carries a risk of damage to the sacral nerves and the deeper pelvic structures. A caudal injection (p 152) is technically easier and achieves effective sacral plexus blockade and should be used in preference to a direct sacral plexus block.

The sciatic nerve can be anaesthetised at a number of points along its course from the greater sciatic foramen to the popliteal fossa. The earliest transgluteal description of Labat is

Figure 2.4
Cutaneous innervation of sciatic nerve

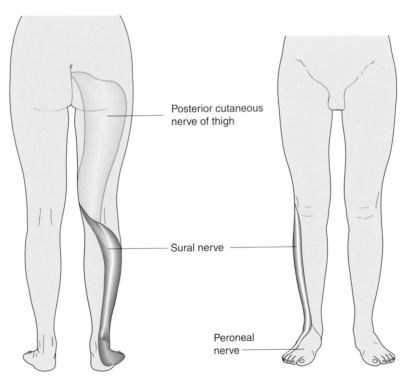

Posterior cutaneous nerve of thigh

Sural nerve

Peroneal nerve

the most proximal and approaches the nerve through the gluteus muscles as it exits the sciatic foramen. A number of posterior, anterior and lateral techniques are described (pp 59–63) which all produce a block at or proximal to a level between the lesser trochanter and ischial tuberosity. There is both a posterior and a lateral approach to the nerve within the popliteal fossa. The proximal approaches produce motor and sensory blockade in both the thigh and the lower leg whereas blockade within the popliteal fossa restricts these effects to the calf and foot only, allowing the patient some control over flexion of the knee.

Since the posterior cutaneous nerve of thigh is so closely associated with the sciatic nerve as they exit the greater sciatic foramen, for all practical purposes, the two nerves are blocked together when proximal sciatic nerve blocks are performed but it will not be blocked with a popliteal fossa approach and the skin of the posterior aspect of the calf will retain sensation, which may be important if a calf tourniquet is applied.

The territories of the five peripheral nerves innervating the hip joint and upper part of the leg overlap considerably and this generally means that multiple nerve blocks are necessary to achieve adequate surgical anaesthesia in a particular field. The sciatic nerve and the femoral nerve are frequently blocked in combination to ensure adequate anaesthesia of the thigh and knee joint. The obturator and the LCNT may also require blockade, depending on the site of surgery, especially for hip joint surgery.

Indications

Hip joint surgery

A lumbar paravertebral or lumbar plexus block can be used (usually in combination with a light general anaesthetic or intravenous sedation) where, for instance a spinal or epidural technique is contraindicated. A '3 in 1' block is not so effective because it does not reliably block the LCNT or the obturator and would not be expected to block the skin overlying the iliac crest and buttock. For complete anaesthesia of the hip joint, a sciatic nerve block is needed in combination with the plexus block and this can be achieved in the lateral position by performing both a psoas compartment block and a 'Labat' approach to the sciatic nerve (pp 54 and 60). In

the frail elderly patient, peripheral nerve blocks, combined with light general anaesthesia can be especially useful in avoiding haemodynamic instability providing that the total volume and concentration of local anaesthetic drug is carefully controlled. A combination of femoral, LCNT and iliac crest blocks is an effective means of providing analgesia for fixation of neck of femur fractures, while a sciatic nerve block will also be needed if a total or hemi-hip arthroplasty is performed.

Knee joint surgery

Femoral and sciatic nerve blocks provide intra-operative and post-operative analgesia for all types of knee surgery. The femoral, sciatic, LCNT and obturator nerves all supply fibres to the joint, either directly or via neural plexuses within the thigh and it may be preferable to consider discrete nerve block of each individual nerve for total anaesthesia of the joint.

Long bone surgery

Femoral nerve and sciatic nerve blocks in combination can be used for surgery to both the femur and the tibia and fibula. To restrict the extent of blockade, popliteal fossa block is effective for surgery to the tibia and fibula.

Trauma

Femoral nerve blocks are indicated in the management of pain following bony or soft tissue injury of the thigh, both in adults and children. Below the knee, sciatic and femoral blocks are equally useful although it is important to consider the risk of compartment syndrome developing within the interosseous compartments and its symptoms being masked by dense nerve blockade.

Skin grafts

The lateral aspect of the thigh is a common donor site for skin grafts. LCNT block is a very good means of providing analgesia to the donor site.

Sympathetic blockade

The major peripheral nerves are accompanied by sympathetic nerve fibres and significant sympathetic nerve blockade results from somatic nerve blocks. This can produce clinically useful vasodilatation for patients with peripheral vascular disease, especially in the management of ischaemic rest pain and pre-gangrenous changes. Prolonged peripheral nerve blocks may also be useful in treating sympathetically maintained chronic pain states. Nerve sheath catheters can be inserted for prolonged femoral and sciatic nerve blocks to improve circulation and treat some chronic pain states (p 127).

The lower leg and foot

The nerve supply to the lower leg and foot

There are three terminal nerves that supply the lower leg, ankle joint and foot – two are terminal components of the sciatic nerve. The third is the saphenous nerve (the terminal sensory branch of the femoral nerve), which contributes a variable area of cutaneous sensation.

- Tibial
  - medial plantar branch
  - lateral plantar branch
  - calcaneal branch
  - sural (arising in popliteal fossa)
- Common peroneal
  - deep peroneal
  - superficial peroneal
- Saphenous
- Digital

Tibial nerve

This descends from the popliteal fossa between the heads of the gastrocnemius muscle, sending motor fibres to the plantar flexor muscles and then passes posterior to the medial malleolus deep to the flexor retinaculum The nerve then divides into the medial and lateral plantar branches, which supply the muscles and deep structures of the sole of the foot and the medial calcaneal nerve that supplies the heel (Figure 2.5).

Medial plantar nerve

The medial plantar nerve innervates the antero-medial surface of the sole and the plantar surface of the medial three and a half-toes.

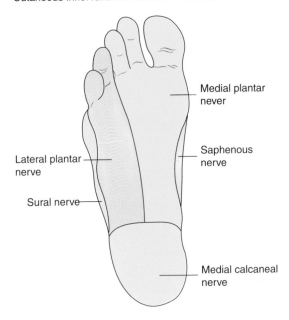

Figure 2.5
Cutaneous innervation of the sole of the foot

Medial plantar never

Saphenous nerve

Lateral plantar nerve

Sural nerve

Medial calcaneal nerve

Lateral plantar nerve

The lateral plantar nerve innervates the antero-lateral surface of the sole and the plantar surface of the lateral one and a half-toes.

Medial calcaneal nerve

The medial calcaneal nerve branches off the tibial nerve behind the medial malleolus and pierces the flexor retinaculum to innervate the skin of the heel and the postero-medial surface of the sole.

Sural nerve

This originates from the tibial nerve in the popliteal fossa and innervates the skin of the postero-lateral aspect of the distal part of the lower leg and then runs between the lateral malleolus and the tendo achilles to supply the skin of the lateral aspect of the ankle joint and heel and the lateral border of the foot and 5th toe.

Common peroneal nerve

The common peroneal is smaller than the tibial nerve and lies lateral to it in the popliteal fossa. The two nerves separate, usually at the apex of the popliteal fossa and the peroneal nerve

Figure 2.6
Cutaneous innervation of superficial peroneal nerve

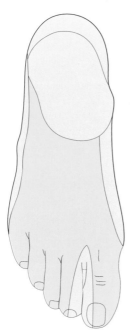

Figure 2.7
Cutaneous innervation of deep peroneal nerve

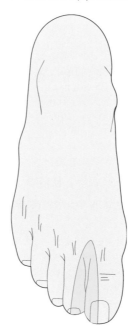

Figure 2.8
Cutaneous innervation of saphenous nerve

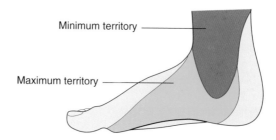

Minimum territory

Maximum territory

follows the medial border of the biceps femoris muscle and tendon until it exits the fossa, passes around the head of the fibula and then divides into the superficial and deep peroneal nerves.

Superficial peroneal nerve

This runs between the peroneus muscles and extensor digitorum longus, pierces the deep fascia in the distal part of the leg and divides into a medial and lateral branch. These supply the skin of the dorsum of the foot, the medial side of the great toe and the dorsal surface of all the toes, except the skin of the 1st web space (deep peroneal) and the lateral side of the 5th toe (sural nerve) (Figure 2.6).

Deep peroneal nerve

The deep peroneal nerve descends with the anterior tibial artery, supplying motor nerves to the dorsiflexors of the foot and articular branches to the ankle and then crosses the front of the ankle joint lateral to the pulse of dorsalis pedis to and supply the bones and joints of the dorsum of the foot and the skin of the 1st web space (Figure 2.7).

Saphenous nerve

The Saphenous nerve (L2, 3, 4) divides into two branches at the level of the medial malleolus, one of which innervates the skin overlying the ankle and the other which continues forward to supply the medial aspect of the foot as far distal as the metatarso-phalangeal joint of the great toe, although the combined territory is variable (Figure 2.8).

Digital nerves

The toes are each innervated by four digital nerves, two dorsal and two ventral. The digital nerves are the terminal branches of the peroneal nerves (dorsally) and the tibial nerve (ventrally). They are formed at the level of the bases of the metatarsals from where they pass distally, closely applied to the periosteum of the bones of each digit.

Applied anatomy of the lower leg

The popliteal fossa is a diamond-shaped structure with its long axis joining the angle between the hamstring muscles proximally and the angle between the heads of gastrocnemius distally. The sciatic nerve divides into its tibial and peroneal component nerves, usually at the point of entry into the fossa at its apex. The nerves are lateral and superficial to the popliteal vessels and can be located using either a posterior or lateral approach. In terms of patient management, the lateral approach is easier as the patient does not need to be positioned prone. The peroneal nerve should never be blocked at the level of the head of the fibula as the nerve is tightly bound within an osteofascial compartment at this point and there is a high risk of damaging the nerve – either by direct needle trauma or with hydrostatic pressure from the local anaesthetic injection.

The saphenous nerve emerges from under the sartorius muscle as it inserts into the tibial plateau on the medial side of the knee. It is usually deep to the long saphenous vein at this point and is easy to block with a deep subcutaneous injection, taking care to avoid damage to the vein.

Applied anatomy around the ankle and foot

All the nerves supplying the foot are all superficial and easy to locate. Despite a reputation for being 'difficult and unpredictable' to block and consequently relatively underused, the approaches (pp 65–68) are highly successful when used regularly. There is also no need to position the patient prone as described in some existing texts and there is little inconvenience for either patient or anaesthetist.

The cutaneous territories of each nerve have a varied distribution and do not correspond with the underlying deeper structures. Therefore, it is always advisable to block adjacent nerves especially if the site of surgery is close to the boundary of a nerve territory. Thus, the sural, the superficial and deep peroneal nerves may need to be blocked to ensure complete anaesthesia at the boundaries of the sole of the foot. Superficial and deep peroneal nerves are invariably blocked in combination because of the overlapping cutaneous territories. One point of needle insertion may be used for both techniques.

Although the saphenous nerve can be blocked at the ankle, it may be more appropriate to use a more proximal technique, for example at the level of the tibial plateau. This is especially suitable if the proposed operation site lies around the medial malleolus. In both approaches the nerve is subcutaneous and is easily blocked by subcutaneous infiltration.

The medial calcaneal and the medial and lateral plantar nerves all pass deep to the flexor retinaculum and thus may all be blocked by a single injection beneath the retinaculum at a point midway between the heel and the sustentaculum tali, which can be palpated as a bony ridge just below the medial malleolus. In most cases, all three branches will be blocked but it is possible for the calcaneal branch to be partially blocked, if too small a volume of local anaesthetic is used.

If the more proximal blocks of the foot are not adequate in providing analgesia to a particular digit, the appropriate digital nerves can be blocked within the web space (p 68) to reinforce the block.

Indications

1. Lower leg surgery including:
   - long bone surgery of the lower leg, for example high tibial osteotomy
   - arthrodesis/fusion of ankle joint
   - tarsal surgery
   - repair tendo achilles

A popliteal nerve block and a saphenous nerve block at the knee are the best combination for extensive surgery (pp 63–64).

2. Ankle joint and foot surgery
   - Bunionectomy/osteotomy of hallux valgus
   - K wiring of toe(s)
   - avulsion of in-growing toenail
   - removal of foreign body
   - trauma to foot
   - amputation of toes/forefoot

For most surgical procedures on the foot, it is not necessary to block more than two or three nerves in combination. If the intended surgery is very extensive, a more proximal approach is appropriate. The sciatic nerve can be blocked in the popliteal fossa and combined if necessary with a saphenous nerve block to provide complete anaesthesia of the lower leg and foot. Alternatively, nerve blockade at the ankle will restrict motor and sensory block to the foot, leaving the extensor and flexor muscles of the lower leg unaffected. This can be of advantage in some forms of foot surgery and allows the patient early post-operative control of the leg whilst maintaining analgesia of the foot.

Peripheral nerve block techniques of the lower extremity

Introduction

Lumbar epidural, spinal or caudal injection techniques have been the mainstay of regional anaesthesia for the lower extremity for many years. They are relatively easy techniques to perform with a high success rate but they are associated with significant complications and are accompanied by the disadvantages of bladder and bowel disturbance and bilateral limb immobility. Increasingly, peripheral nerve block techniques are being used and can offer the advantages of long-lasting intra- and post-operative analgesia, improved mobility and a lower profile of side effects and complications when compared to systemic opioid analgesics and central neural blockade.

Lumbar plexus block

The traditional approach to the lumbar plexus is paravertebral and the original descriptions are based on multiple injections – one at each lumbar transverse process (Figure 2.9). More recent techniques have been described which only require a single needle insertion at either the L2, 3 or L3, 4 interspaces. There is controversy about the precise mode of action of these techniques, especially where large volumes of local anaesthetic are used, as the local anaesthetic may flow medially into the epidural space and produce most of its effects as an epidural block.

Lumbar paravertebral block

Surface landmarks Spinous processes of lumbar vertebrae.
Patient position Either (i) prone over a pillow placed under the abdomen or (ii) in the lateral position with the injected side uppermost.

Figure 2.9
Approaches to the lumbar plexus

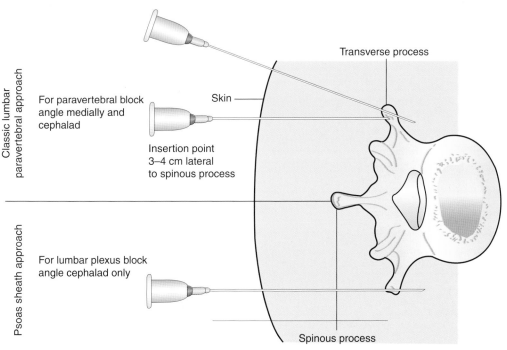

Classic lumbar paravertebral approach

For paravertebral block angle medially and cephalad

Insertion point 3–4 cm lateral to spinous process

Skin

Transverse process

Psoas sheath approach

For lumbar plexus block angle cephalad only

Spinous process

Technique The technique is the same whichever patient position is used. Identify the spinous processes and mark a point 3 cm lateral to the cephalad edge of the third lumbar spine and insert an 8 cm 22G spinal needle perpendicular to the skin until the transverse process is contacted, This usually occurs at a depth of 4–5 cm, at which point, withdraw the needle slightly and re-angle it both cephalad and medially (about 25–30° to the midline). Advance the needle slowly so that it just passes cephalad to the proximal edge of the transverse process. Approximately 2 cm deep to the transverse process, paraesthesiae will be elicited in the distribution of the L2 nerve root. After careful aspiration to ensure that cerebro-spinal fluid or blood is not present, inject 20–30 ml of local anaesthetic. A dilute solution will suffice because the local anaesthetic is applied directly to the nerve roots.

Agent	Concn (%)	Volume (ml)	Onset (min)	Dur (h)
l-bupiv	0.25	20–30	45	4

Figure 2.10
Psoas compartment block

The psoas compartment (sheath) block (Figure 2.10)

Surface landmarks Spinous processes of 3rd or 4th lumbar vertebrae.
Patient position Left or right lateral, with side to be blocked uppermost.
Technique Use a skin marker to identify the 3rd lumbar spinous process and draw a perpendicular line 5 cm lateral from the spinous process (a). The end of this line should intersect a line drawn parallel to the lumbar spine, starting at the posterior superior iliac spine. Mark a point 3 cm caudad along this line – this is the needle insertion point, which should lie directly over the transverse process of L4 (b). These measurements are typical for an adult male but in small adults, 5 cm laterally may result in missing the transverse process and 3.5–4 cm is a more suitable distance.

Use a 100–150 mm long insulated needle, according to the patient's body mass, and insert it perpendicular to the skin making sure that it is kept strictly parallel to the midline (c). Having contacted the transverse process of L4,

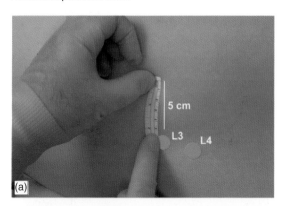

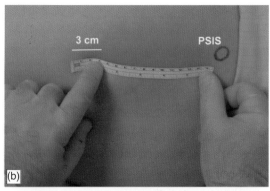

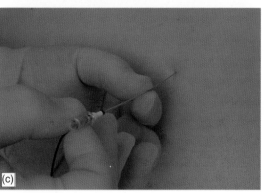

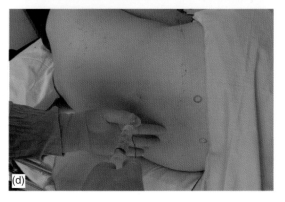

withdraw the needle and re-angle it either cephalad or caudad, keeping it in a plane parallel to the midline and advance it no more than 2 cm beyond the transverse process (d). The total distance from the skin should be no more than 8–9 cm unless the patient has a large body mass index. Entry into the psoas compartment is confirmed by using peripheral nerve stimulator to produce pulse-synchronous movement of the quadriceps mechanism of the thigh. After negative aspiration for blood, inject 25–35 ml of solution. The duration of a psoas compartment block is relatively short because of the redistribution and absorption of local anaesthetic within the muscle compartment. The block can be prolonged for surgery and post-operative analgesia by inserting an indwelling catheter (p 128).

The original description of this technique is based on an identical procedure but is performed using the spinous process of L4 and the transverse process of L5. Access may be more difficult at this point of entry as the iliac crest may interfere with needle access.

Psoas compartment blocks are easily combined with the classical Labat sciatic nerve block (p 60) for hip surgery, as the patient position is the same for both techniques.

Agent	Concn (%)	Volume (ml)	Onset (min)	Dur (h)
l-bupiv	0.25	35–40	20	3–5
l-bupiv	0.5	25–30	20	4–8

Distal approach to the lumbar plexus

In 1973 Alon Winnie described a distal approach to the lumbar plexus, using the same landmarks and technique as for the femoral nerve block. It is popularly referred to as the '3 in 1' block, because it is intended to produce a combined block of the femoral, obturator and LCNT, using a large volume of local anaesthetic – up to 30 ml.

The three nerves are not always reliably blocked even if large volumes of local anaesthetic are injected by this distal approach. The obturator is most frequently missed due to its more medial and deep anatomical course. The LCNT may also be missed as it arises more proximally than the other two nerves. Conversely, because the lumbar plexus contains a major contribution to the sacral plexus – the lumbosacral trunk, a '3 in 1' block may spill over into the sciatic nerve distribution. This block can vary from a '1 in 1' to a '4 in 1' block depending on the volume of local anaesthetic solution injected and anatomical variation within the psoas compartment.

Research using CT scanning indicates that the spread of local anaesthetic in a successful '3 in 1' block may not be proximal and retrograde, following the femoral nerve within its sheath as commonly understood. It may actually produce blockade of the three nerves at a peripheral level by spreading medially and laterally, under the ilio-pectineal fascia from the point of injection and remaining distal to the inguinal ligament. Other evidence suggests that if an indwelling catheter is inserted into the femoral nerve sheath, it may well pass easily into the psoas compartment and therefore produce a block of the lumbar plexus. There may well be a distinct difference between the distal approach to the lumbar plexus using a catheter which produces a true plexus block and a single-shot injection at the level of the femoral nerve which blocks the three terminal nerves by peripheral spread of local anaesthetic.

Femoral nerve block

Surface landmarks Inguinal ligament, femoral artery.
Patient position Supine with the lower limb slightly abducted.
Technique Mark the inguinal ligament by drawing a line between the ASIS and the pubic tubercle. Palpate the femoral artery pulse and mark a point approximately 1 cm lateral to the pulse and 1–2 cm below the inguinal ligament. Insert a 22G short bevel 50 mm insulated needle at this mark and slowly advance it, aiming cephalad at an angle of about 45° to the skin in a plane parallel to the midline (Figure 2.11). If the bevel of the needle is placed flat on the skin, a greater degree of 'feel' will help to identify two distinct 'pops' as the tip of the needle penetrates firstly the fascia lata and then the ilio-pectineal fascia that invests the nerve (Figure 2.12). Depending on the amount of superficial fat, the nerve is between 1 and 3 cm deep to the skin. A peripheral nerve stimulator will assist accurate needle placement because the nerve divides into its anterior and posterior divisions as it emerges distal to the inguinal ligament. It is important to identify branches of the posterior division, which supply motor innervation of the thigh muscles and sensory innervation of the majority

of the knee joint synovium and cartilage. It also gives rise to the saphenous nerve. The nerve stimulator should produce pulse-synchronous movement of the rectus femoris, vastus medialis and vastus lateralis muscles so that the patella is clearly seen to move. Pulse-synchronous movement of the sartorius muscle indicates that the anterior division of the nerve is being stimulated and anaesthesia of the thigh and knee joint will be unreliable as the anterior division supplies only a limited area of skin. In view of the close proximity of the femoral vessels, careful aspiration of the syringe is essential prior to injection.

Figure 2.11
Femoral nerve block

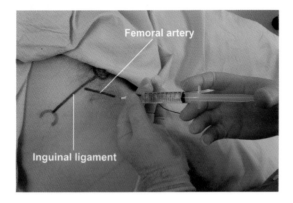

Agent	Concn (%)	Volume (ml)	Onset (min)	Dur (h)
l-bupiv	0.5	10–15	30	8–12
ropiv	1.0	10–15	20	12–24
For a '3 in 1' block				
l-bupiv	0.5	30	30	8–12
ropiv	0.75	30	30	8–10

Figure 2.12
Femoral nerve block, anatomy

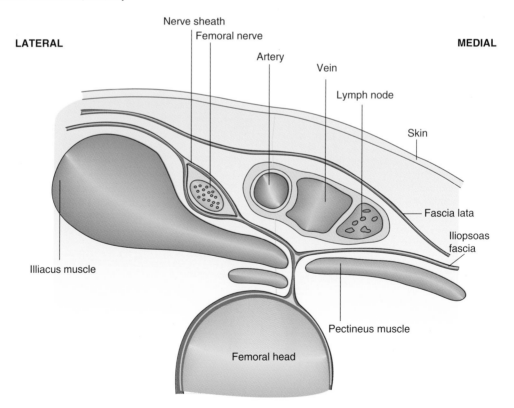

Obturator nerve block

The obturator nerve has the reputation of being difficult to block, with a low success rate and few indications. The 'classic' description of the technique is rather difficult and uncomfortable for the conscious patient, as it requires repeated identification of the bony landmarks, which define the obturator canal. However, the 'Figure of four' approach is easy to perform and has a high success rate, especially if a peripheral nerve stimulator is used.

'Classical' approach

Surface landmarks Pubic tubercle, superior ramus of pelvis.
Patient position Supine with the leg slightly abducted.
Technique Palpate the pubic tubercle and raise a skin wheal approximately 1–2 cm inferior and 1–2 cm lateral to the tubercle. Insert an 8 cm 22G spinal needle in a cephalad and slightly medial direction, as in Figure 2.13a, until the lateral aspect of the pubis is contacted. Withdraw the needle slightly and re-direct it laterally towards the ASIS retaining the same angle to the skin (Figure 2.13b). Usually the needle contacts the superior pubic ramus just above the obturator canal, although the needle may directly enter the canal. If the ramus is identified, re-angle the needle by raising the hub and directing it inferiorly until the obturator canal is entered (this will be felt as a slight resistance followed by a 'give' when the needle penetrates the obturator membrane).

Limited and variable cutaneous innervation means that paraesthesiae may not be elicited in the conscious patient and a peripheral nerve stimulator will give a more accurate location by producing pulse-synchronous movement of the adductor muscles. Inject the solution after aspiration.

Figure 2.13a and b
Obturator nerve block, 'classical approach'

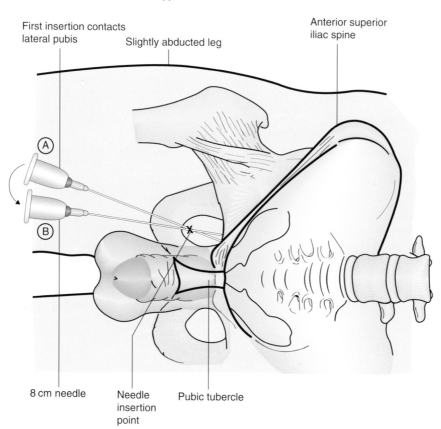

First insertion contacts lateral pubis

Slightly abducted leg

Anterior superior iliac spine

A

B

8 cm needle

Needle insertion point

Pubic tubercle

Agent	Concn (%)	Volume (ml)	Onset (min)	Dur (h)
l-bupiv	0.5	10	20	6–12
ropiv	0.75	10	15	12–18

'Figure of four' approach

Surface landmarks Insertion of the adductor muscle tendons into the pubis.

Patient position Supine with the sole of the foot of the leg to blocked against the medial side of the knee of the other leg to make the 'Figure of four' position (Figure 2.14).

Technique Identify the insertion of the adductor magnus and the adductor brevis muscles into the pubis. Raise a skin wheal over the gap between the tendons about 1 cm inferior to the pubis (Figure 2.15). Insert a 100 cm insulated needle in the horizontal plane aiming towards the ipsilateral ASIS. The needle will penetrate

the obturator membrane covering the obturator foramen, often with a slight but definite 'pop', at a depth of about 5 cm and pulse-synchronous stimulation of the adductor muscles occurs at this point. After aspiration, inject 5–6 ml of solution. The needle will directly enter the foramen in the majority of cases but if the bony boundaries of the foramen are encountered withdraw the needle slightly and re-direct appropriately.

The advantage of the Figure of four approach is that needle insertion is in a single, consistent direction which places the needle tip close to the division of the nerve into its two branches, an important factor in achieving complete block of the motor and cutaneous distribution.

Agent	Concn (%)	Volume (ml)	Onset (min)	Dur (h)
l-bupiv	0.5	5–7	20	6–12
ropiv	0.75	5–7	20	8–12

LCNT block

Surface landmarks ASIS, Inguinal ligament, fascia lata.

Patient position Supine.

Technique Palpate the ASIS to define the insertion of the inguinal ligament. Insert a 3.5 cm short bevelled needle 2–3 cm caudad to the spine and 2–3 cm medial, as in Figure 2.16. Just deep to the subcutaneous tissue the fascia lata is felt as a definite resistance to the needle and if the needle is moved slightly each way in the horizontal plane, the fascia can be 'scratched'. Advance the needle through the fascia with a

Figure 2.14
Obturator nerve block, 'Figure of four' position

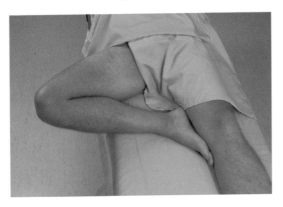

Figure 2.15
Obturator nerve block

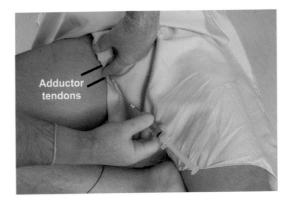

Adductor tendons

Figure 2.16
Lateral cutaneous nerve of the thigh block

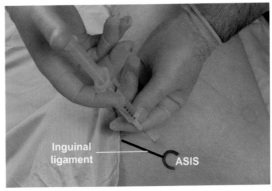

Inguinal ligament

ASIS

definite 'pop' and inject 10 ml of solution immediately deep to the fascia (Figure 2.16).

The nerve can also be blocked by an approach above the inguinal ligament but the end point is more difficult to identify and this is therefore not recommended.

Agent	Concn (%)	Volume (ml)	Onset (min)	Dur (h)
l-bupiv	0.5	10	20	4–6

Iliac crest block

Although the subcostal nerve (T12) is not a branch of the lumbar plexus, the lateral cutaneous branch of this nerve supplies the skin over the iliac crest and proximal aspect of the hip. It therefore needs to be blocked if peripheral nerve blocks are used to provide analgesia for hip surgery. It can be difficult to block at the level of the twelfth rib in the obese or immobile patient and is more easily approached at the iliac crest.

Figure 2.17
Iliac crest block, lateral view

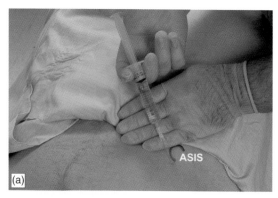

(a)

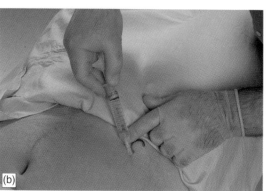

(b)

Surface landmarks ASIS, iliac crest.
Patient position Supine.
Technique Make a subcutaneous injection of local anaesthetic from the ASIS posteriorly to the midpoint of the iliac crest using an 8 cm 22G spinal needle (Figure 2.17).

Agent	Concn (%)	Volume (ml)	Onset (min)	Dur (h)
l-bupiv	0.5	10	20	8
lido	1	10	10	4

The sciatic plexus block

The sciatic plexus is relatively inaccessible to a direct approach due to its protection by the anterior surface of the sacrum and ilium. Conventionally, central neural blockade (see caudal block, p 152) is used to block the sacral nerve roots within the sacral canal before they emerge to form the plexus. Discrete blockade of the plexus by a series of injections through the dorsal sacral foraminae has been described but this is a difficult and unreliable technique and it carries a relatively high risk of nerve damage within the sacral foraminae. Proximal approaches to the sciatic nerve will produce a degree of retrograde spread to the plexus, sufficient for lower extremity blockade.

Sciatic nerve block

The sciatic nerve is the largest and most deeply situated peripheral nerve; it is approximately 2.5 cm wide as it emerges from the greater sciatic foramen and between 5 and 10 cm deep to the skin (depending on the particular technique used). In the conscious patient, sciatic nerve blocks can be uncomfortable and difficult to perform and it is usual to offer sedation or a light general anaesthetic to the patient before performing the block. In both conscious and anaesthetised patients, the use of a nerve stimulator will improve the accuracy of nerve location and therefore ensure a higher success rate. Due to the size and depth of the nerve, it is important to use a high concentration of local anaesthetic (0.75% ropivacaine and *l*-bupivacaine or 2% lidocaine) and to allow plenty of time for the block to develop. It may take 45–60 min for full motor and sensory block to occur.

Figure 2.18
Sciatic nerve block, classical transgluteal approach

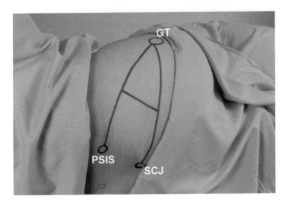

There are four proximal approaches to the sciatic nerve – two posterior (transgluteal and lithotomy) one anterior and one lateral. A more distal approach within the popliteal fossa blocks the terminal branches of the sciatic nerve – the tibial and common peroneal nerves.

Transgluteal posterior approach (Labat)

Surface landmarks Posterior superior iliac spine, sacro-coccygeal joint (SCJ), greater trochanter (GT).
Patient position Lateral position, with the side to be blocked uppermost. Extend the bottom leg and flex the top leg to 90°.
Technique Use a skin-marking pen to draw a line from the highest prominence of the greater trochanter to the posterior superior iliac spine. Draw a second line from the same point of reference on the greater trochanter to the sacro-coccygeal joint (or just below the sacral hiatus if the joint is difficult to locate). Draw a third line at 90° from the midpoint of the first line to intersect the second line; this intersection overlies the point at which the sciatic nerve emerges from the sciatic foramen (Figure 2.18). Insert an 80 or 100 mm 22G insulated needle through the point of intersection, perpendicular to the skin surface and advance through the gluteal muscles. If you touch bone at a depth of 5–6 cm (deeper in a large patient), withdraw the needle slightly and re-direct it in a systematic way until it passes into the sciatic foramen. At this point, a peripheral nerve stimulator should indicate close proximity to the nerve by characteristic movements of the lower leg and foot. The nerve is usually found at a depth of 6–8 cm in a patient of medium build. Paraesthesiae are most likely to be elicited in the

lateral (peroneal) component of the nerve, that is on the lateral aspect of the shin or the dorsum of the foot and nerve stimulation produces dorsiflexion and eversion of the foot. Stimulation of the larger tibial component will induce plantarflexion and inversion of the foot. Providing that the identification is unequivocal, 15–20 ml of local anaesthetic is injected without further needle re-positioning to locate the other nerve component.

Agent	Concn (%)	Volume (ml)	Onset (min)	Dur (h)
l-bupiv	0.75	10–15	30	12–18
ropiv	0.75	15–20	30	12–18

Posterior lithotomy approach (Figure 2.19)

Due to the importance of correct patient positioning, this approach may be unsuitable for patients with lower limb trauma or advanced joint disease.
Surface landmarks Greater trochanter, ischial tuberosity (IT).
Patient position Supine, with an assistant holding the leg to be blocked flexed to 90° at both the hip and the knee.
Technique Draw a line between the greater trochanter and the ischial tuberosity (a) and identify the midpoint. In thin, muscular limbs you will usually be able to see or palpate the intermuscular groove between the hamstring (biceps femoris and semitendinosus) muscles and the midpoint of your line will normally overlie this groove. Insert a 100 mm insulated needle approximately 1 cm above the midpoint of this line, perpendicular to the skin (b). The needle passes through the intermuscular septum of the hamstrings and the nerve lies between 5 and 7 cm deep to the skin. If bony contact is made, withdraw the needle 2–3 cm and re-angle slightly medially to place the needle tip medial to the lesser trochanter. A peripheral nerve stimulator should be used to locate the nerve, starting stimulation at about 4 cm depth. Initially, you will see direct stimulation of the hamstrings producing flexion of the knee but as the needle is advanced pulse-synchronous movement of the calf muscles and the foot occurs as the needle approaches either the peroneal or the tibial component of the sciatic nerve (refer to classical sciatic approach for details of foot

Figure 2.19
Sciatic nerve block, lithotomy approach

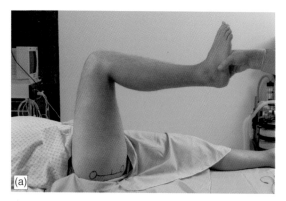

(a)

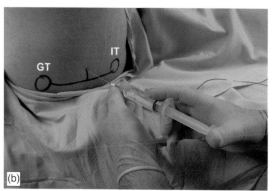

(b)

Figure 2.20
Sciatic nerve block, anterior approach

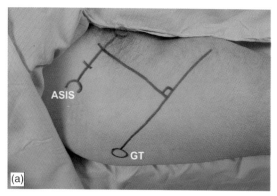

(a)

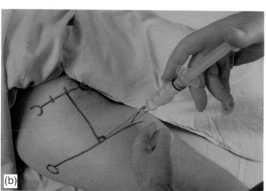

(b)

movements). Following satisfactory location of the nerve inject 15–20 ml of local anaesthetic.

The lithotomy approach is easy to learn as the nerve is at its most superficial and the landmarks are readily identified even in the obese leg. The main drawbacks are the need for assistance in supporting the leg during the procedure and the difficulty in positioning patients with painful joints.

Agent	Concn (%)	Volume (ml)	Onset (min)	Dur (h)
l-bupiv	0.75	15–20	30	12–18

Anterior approach (Figure 2.20)

Surface landmarks Inguinal ligament, prominence of greater trochanter.
Patient position Supine with leg slightly abducted and internally rotated.
Technique Draw a line along the inguinal ligament and divide it into equal thirds,

marking the junction of the middle and medial thirds. Draw a line from the prominence of the greater trochanter parallel to the inguinal ligament across the anterior surface of the thigh. Draw a perpendicular line from the junction of the medial and middle thirds to intersect the parallel line (a). Insert a 100–150 mm insulated needle at the point of intersection, perpendicular to the skin – because of the curvature of the thigh the needle will be advanced in a dorso-lateral direction passing medial to the lesser trochanter as shown in (b). Use a nerve stimulator to confirm nerve location once the needle has been advanced to a depth of 8–10 cm, depending on the size of the thigh. The sciatic nerve lies just deep to the lesser trochanter in a fascial space behind adductor magnus and it is common to touch bone as the needle advances. If this happens, note the depth at which bone is reached and withdraw the needle slightly and re-angle more medially. It may also help to internally rotate the leg more in order to rotate the lesser trochanter posteriorly and expose the sciatic nerve to the advancing needle. The nerve is usually 2.5–3 cm deep to the lesser trochanter as the needle is re-introduced. After locating the nerve, aspirate to check for intravascular needle placement and then slowly inject 15–20 ml of local anaesthetic.

The depth of this approach and the muscle bulk traversed by the needle makes this a more difficult technique than other approaches and can be painful for a conscious patient. Consider using intravenous sedation or a light general anaesthetic before performing the block. The main benefit of the anterior approach is that the patient does not need to be moved and this makes it suitable for patients with lower limb trauma, advanced joint disease and patients who will not tolerate being turned into the lateral position.

Agent	Concn (%)	Volume (ml)	Onset (min)	Dur (h)
l-bupiv	0.75	10–15	up to 60	12–24
ropiv	0.75	10–15	up to 60	12–18
lido	2	10–20	45	8–12

Lateral approach (Figure 2.21)

Surface landmarks Prominence of the greater trochanter.
Patient position Supine with the leg slightly internally rotated and supported with a pillow under the foot and calf.
Technique Palpate the prominence of the greater trochanter and then mark the inferior margin of the greater trochanter. Draw a 5 cm line distally from the inferior margin along the axis of the femur (a). Insert a 100–150 mm insulated needle perpendicularly to the skin and advance until it touches the femur (b). Note the depth at which the needle touches the femur, withdraw the needle a few cm and re-direct the angle of needle insertion posteriorly so that as you advance the needle again, it passes posterior to the femur. At a depth of 8–12 cm, the peripheral nerve stimulator will produce pulse-synchronous movement of the calf muscles or foot – usually in the common peroneal distribution of the nerve due to the lateral approach of the needle. Inject 15–20 ml of local anaesthetic after negative aspiration.

The lateral approach requires a larger volume of local anaesthetic in order to block the more medial tibial component of the sciatic nerve and may be less reliable than other techniques. It has the advantages of not having to move the patient and that the landmarks may be easier to locate than more proximal approaches in obese patients.

Agent	Concn (%)	Volume (ml)	Onset (min)	Dur (h)
l-bupiv	0.5	15–20	45	12–18
ropiv	0.75	15–20	45	12–14

Distal nerve blocks of the lower limb

Distal nerve blocks for the lower leg can be performed at both the knee and the ankle. At the knee, the terminal branches of the sciatic nerve can be blocked within the popliteal fossa and the saphenous nerve can be blocked on the

Figure 2.21
Landmarks for lateral approach to sciatic nerve/needle insertion for lateral approach to sciatic nerve

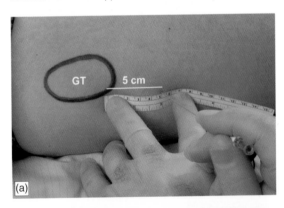

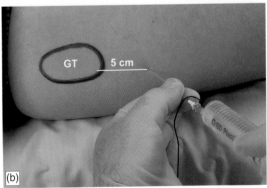

medial aspect of the knee joint. A combination of these nerve blocks will produce complete anaesthesia/analgesia of the lower leg and foot, leaving the motor and sensory supply to the thigh unaffected. This retains useful muscle function in the proximal part of the lower extremity, which is advantageous in short-stay surgery.

Saphenous nerve block

Surface landmarks Medial condyle of tibia, tibial tuberosity.

Patient position Supine with the leg externally rotated.

Technique Identify the bony prominence of the tibial tuberosity and palpate the bony surface of the medial tibial condyle at the level of the tuberosity. The saphenous nerve is in the deep subcutaneous tissue at this level, usually deep to the long saphenous vein. Insert a 22G 80 mm spinal needle 2 cm postero-medial to the tibial tuberosity as in Figure 2.22 keeping in the deep subcutaneous plane. Inject as the needle is advanced along the medial border of the condyle and aspirate frequently to avoid injecting into the saphenous vein. Alternatively, if the vein is easily visible, deposit the local anaesthetic volume in divided doses either side of the vein as the nerve is usually close to the vein.

Agent	Concn (%)	Volume (ml)	Onset (min)	Dur (h)
l-bupiv	0.5	10–15	15	6–8

Figure 2.22
Saphenous nerve block

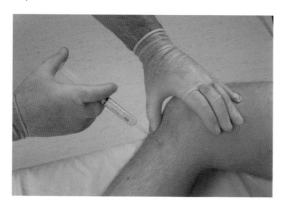

Popliteal fossa block

The two principle terminal branches (peroneal and tibial nerves) of the sciatic nerve can be blocked by a single injection into the popliteal fossa. For complete anaesthesia below the knee, a combined technique with a saphenous nerve block at the knee (see above) is necessary. Popliteal fossa block is easy to perform, especially with a peripheral nerve stimulator, using either the posterior or the lateral approach.

Posterior approach (Figure 2.23)

Surface landmarks Posterior skin crease of knee joint, biceps femoris tendon (lateral side of knee), semitendinosis tendon (medial side of knee).

Patient position Prone with the lower leg and foot supported on a pillow.

Technique Define the boundaries of the popliteal fossa by marking the tendons of the hamstring muscles and the posterior skin crease of the knee joint, which should then form a triangle with the skin crease as the base and the proximal end of the fossa as the apex. From the midpoint of the baseline draw a perpendicular line to the apex of the triangle (a). The needle insertion point is 5–6 cm proximal to the baseline and 1 cm lateral to this line. Insert a 50 mm 22G short bevel needle, angled slightly cephalad and advance 2–3 cm, taking care to avoid intravascular placement by keeping the needle lateral to the vertical line (b). In a large knee, the nerves may lie up to 4 cm deep. Use a peripheral nerve stimulator to evoke either peroneal or tibial pulse-synchronous stimulation and after aspiration, inject 20–25 ml of solution. There should be little resistance to the flow of solution.

Agent	Concn (%)	Volume (ml)	Onset (min)	Dur (h)
l-bupiv	0.5	20–25	20	6–12

Lateral approach (Figure 2.24)

Surface landmarks Upper pole of the patella, border of vastus lateralis, biceps femoris tendon.

Patient position Supine, with the knee flexed to 10–20°.

Figure 2.23
Popliteal fossa block posterior approach

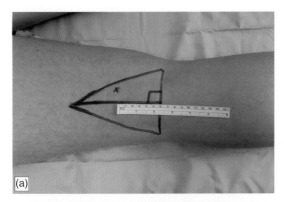

(a)

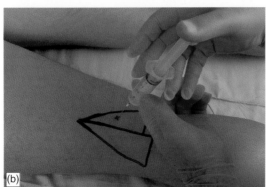

(b)

Figure 2.24
Landmarks and needle insertion for the lateral approach to the popliteal fossa

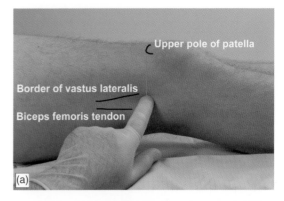

Upper pole of patella

Border of vastus lateralis

Biceps femoris tendon

(a)

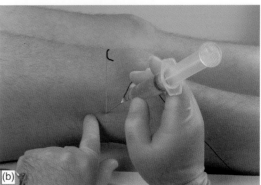

(b)

Technique With the knee slightly flexed, to relax the muscles and tendons of the joint, palpate the upper pole of the patella and draw a line laterally so that it crosses the lateral border of vastus lateralis and the tendon of biceps femoris. Between these two structures, you should be able to feel an obvious groove (a). Insert an insulated 100 mm needle aiming the needle cephalad 30° and posteriorly (dorsally) 30–40° (b). Advance the needle slowly posterior to the femur and at a depth of 3–4 cm you will observe pulse-synchronous movement of the foot. Normally you will stimulate the peroneal nerve first, as this lies immediately medial to the biceps femoris tendon. Occasionally the needle will advance more medially and stimulate the tibial nerve at a deeper level. By carefully advancing and re-angling the needle it is possible to identify both nerves and anaesthetise each separately with an injection of 10–12 ml to each nerve. It is not necessary to locate each nerve, however, and a single injection of 20–25 ml will be sufficient, once one of the nerves has been located.

Intra-articular block of the knee

The increasing use of arthroscopic knee surgery has led to the development of intra-articular anaesthesia, which is effective both for surgery and post-operative analgesia. There is evidence that the intra-articular injection of morphine and clonidine improves the quality of analgesia following surgery, highlighting the role of peripheral opioid and alpha-2 receptors in inflamed synovial tissue.
Surface landmarks Medial border of patella.
Patient position Supine with knee flexed.
Technique Identify the gap between the medial border of the patella at its distal margin and the medial femoral condyle. There is usually a palpable depression at this point. Insert a 22G short bevel needle into the knee joint, as in Figure 2.25, taking care to avoid damaging the

Figure 2.25
Intra-articular block of the knee

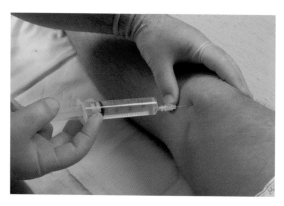

articular surfaces. Inject up to 30 ml of 0.5% *l*-bupivacaine with 1:200,000 adrenaline into the joint (paying regard to the recommended maximum dose). After gentle manipulation of the knee, leave the patient resting for a minimum of 20 min. The addition of 1–2 mg of morphine or 2 mcg/ml of clonidine to the local anaesthetic solution has been shown to prolong post-operative analgesia. Immediately prior to surgery, the portals of entry for the surgical instruments should be infiltrated using 1% lidocaine. The surgeon usually undertakes this, as they can place the local anaesthetic where they wish to introduce the instruments. The benefits of this technique are most apparent in day surgery because there is neither cutaneous sensory deficit nor motor weakness and thus the patient can ambulate immediately after the operation. Provided that sufficient time is allowed for the local anaesthetic solution to penetrate the synovium and for the adrenaline to produce full vasoconstriction, relatively major surgery, including meniscectomy, chondroplasty and synovial resection is possible.

Agent	Concn (%)	Volume (ml)	Onset (min)	Dur (h)
l-bupiv + adren	0.5	30	45	3–5

Ankle and foot

The tibial, superficial and deep peroneal, saphenous and sural nerves can be blocked at the level of the ankle to provide extensive anaesthesia of the foot. The digital nerves of the foot can be blocked at the level of the metatarsals or more distally within the web space.

Tibial nerve block

There are two approaches to the tibial nerve at the level of the medial malleolus. Both are easy to do and have a high success rate in blocking the whole of the sole of the foot. However the 'classical' approach depends on being able to palpate the pulse of the posterior tibial artery in order to find the neurovascular bundle behind the medial malleolus. The pulse may be absent or difficult to palpate in patients with vascular insufficiency or peripheral oedema in which case the sustentaculum tali approach is more reliable and successful as it relies purely on bony landmarks to define the needle insertion point.

'Classical' approach

Surface landmarks Medial malleolus, tibial artery pulsation, periosteum of calcaneum.
Patient position Supine with the leg externally rotated.
Technique Palpate the pulsation of the posterior tibial artery and from a point immediately behind the medial malleolus, insert a 22G short bevel needle parallel to the tibia as in Figure 2.26, towards the palpating finger and deep to the pulsation. The conscious patient will usually feel paraesthesiae just prior to the needle striking the periosteum of the calcaneum. Ensure that the needle tip is not sub-periosteal by withdrawing 2 mm.

Agent	Concn (%)	Volume (ml)	Onset (min)	Dur (h)
l-bupiv	0.5	6	20	6–12
lido	1	6	10	3–4

Sustentaculum tali approach

Surface landmarks Sustentaculum tali, medial border of calcaneum, medial retinaculum of the ankle joint.
Patient position Supine, with the leg externally rotated and the knee flexed slightly.
Technique Identify the medial malleolus and the medial border of the calcaneum. A ridge of

bone, the sustentaculum tali, can then be palpated approximately midway between these two bony landmarks. Insert a 22G short bevel needle perpendicular to the skin over the sustentaculum tali (Figure 2.27) and advance gently through the medial retinaculum (which may be felt as a 'pop') and lightly touch periosteum. The patient may feel paraesthesiae but the injection can be made without this sign, after negative aspiration. Injection should be easy with little resistance to flow. A subcutaneous swelling indicates that the retinaculum has not been penetrated and the needle should be re-positioned more deeply.

Agent	Concn (%)	Volume (ml)	Onset (min)	Dur (h)
l-bupiv	0.5	6–8	20	6–12
lido	1	8	5	3–4

Figure 2.26
Tibial nerve block (classical approach)

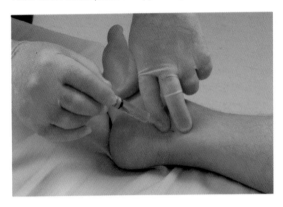

Figure 2.27
Tibial nerve block (Sustentaculum tali approach)

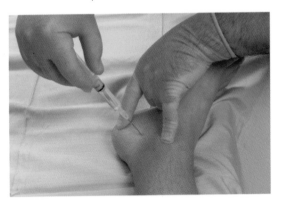

Sural nerve block

Surface landmarks Tendo achilles, lateral malleolus.
Patient position Supine with the leg internally rotated and foot inverted.
Technique Insert a 22G short bevel needle behind the superior border of the lateral malleolus aiming for the lateral border of the tendo achilles as in Figure 2.28. Inject a subcutaneous 'sausage' of local anaesthetic whilst advancing the needle towards the tendo achilles. The nerve has usually divided into several branches at this level and a total of 5 ml of solution is normally sufficient to block all branches.

Agent	Concn (%)	Volume (ml)	Onset (min)	Dur (h)
l-bupiv	0.5	5	20	6–12
lido	1	5	5	3–4

Saphenous nerve block

Surface landmarks Medial malleolus, long saphenous vein.
Patient position Supine with the leg externally rotated and the foot everted.
Technique Identify the long saphenous vein, using venous occlusion to bring it into prominence if necessary. At a point 1 cm proximal and 1 cm anterior to the medial malleolus, inject 5 ml of solution in a subcutaneous infiltration around the vein. Avoid intravenous injection.

Figure 2.28
Sural nerve block

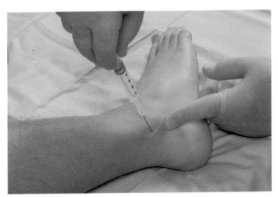

Agent	Concn (%)	Volume (ml)	Onset (min)	Dur (h)
l-bupiv	0.5	3–5	20	6–12
lido	1	3–5	5	3–4

Agent	Concn (%)	Volume (ml)	Onset (min)	Dur (h)
l-bupiv	0.5	5	20	6–12
lido	1	5	5	3

Deep peroneal nerve block

This is almost invariably combined with the superficial peroneal nerve block, as they are performed through the same needle insertion point and are complementary blocks for the dorsum of the foot.

Surface landmarks Intermalleolar skin crease, extensor hallucis longus tendon, dorsalis pedis pulsation.

Patient position Supine with the foot in the neutral position.

Technique At the level of the intermalleolar skin crease across the dorsum of the foot, the dorsalis pedis pulse is palpated between the extensor hallucis longus tendon medially and the extensor digitorum longus tendons laterally and the nerve is between the artery and extensor hallucis longus tendon. With the foot supported in slight extension, insert a 23-G needle just medial to the pulsation of the dorsalis pedis as in Figure 2.29. Advance the needle 1 cm toward the distal end of the tibia. Lightly touch periosteum and then withdraw the needle slightly (to avoid sub-periosteal injection). Inject 3–5 ml of local anaesthetic. If there is resistance to injection, this may indicate that the needle is in a tendon or tendon sheath; withdraw and re-position.

Superficial peroneal nerve

Surface landmarks As for deep peroneal nerve.
Patient position As for deep peroneal nerve.
Technique After completion of the deep peroneal block, withdraw the needle to the subcutaneous tissues and re-angle it laterally. Inject a 5–7 ml 'sausage' of solution as the needle is advanced laterally along a line parallel to the intermalleolar line (Figure 2.30).

Agent	Concn (%)	Volume (ml)	Onset (min)	Dur (h)
l-bupiv	0.5	5–7	20	6–12
lido	1	5	5	3

Metatarsal block

Metatarsal block is useful when anaesthesia of the intrinsic muscles and other deep structures of the forefoot is required in addition to cutaneous analgesia of the toes.

Surface landmarks Inter-metatarsal spaces on dorsum of foot.

Patient position Supine with the foot in the neutral position.

Technique Identify the spaces between the metatarsals corresponding to the toes to be

Figure 2.29
Deep peroneal nerve block

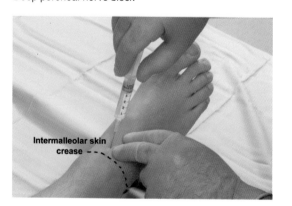

Intermalleolar skin crease

Figure 2.30
Superficial peroneal nerve block

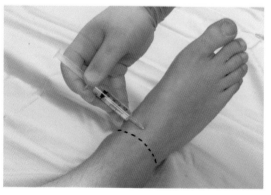

Figure 2.31
Metatarsal block

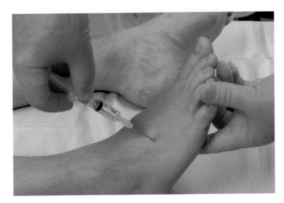

Figure 2.32
Digital nerve block

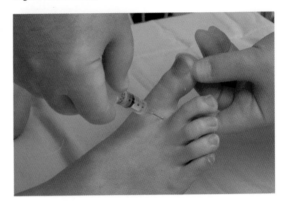

blocked at the midpoint of the metatarsal bones
(halfway down the dorsum of the foot). Insert a
22G short bevel needle vertically downwards
aiming towards the plantar surface of the foot.
Place a palpating finger on the sole to detect the
needle approaching the deep plantar fascia, as
shown in Figure 2.31. The needle should not
penetrate the plantar fascia as the digital nerves
lie above it. Inject 2 ml of solution, withdraw the
needle slowly while a injecting a further 2 ml
and finally inject 2 ml at the level of the dorsal
surface of the metatarsal bone.

Agent	Concn (%)	Volume (ml)	Onset (min)	Dur (h)
l-bupiv	0.5	6	20	6–12
lido	1	6	5–10	3–4

Digital nerve block

The digital nerves can be blocked at the level of
the metatarso-phalangeal joints either side of
the appropriate toe(s) when anaesthesia/
analgesia is restricted just to the toes.
Surface landmarks Metatarso-phalangeal joints,
web spaces.
Patient position Supine with the foot in neutral
position.
Technique Insert a 23G hypodermic needle
vertically downwards at a point above the web
space, just distal to the M-P joint, as in Figure
2.32. Place a finger under the plantar surface of
the web space to detect the approaching needle
tip as it reaches the plantar border of the
proximal phalanx. Withdraw the needle slowly

Figure 2.33
Web space block

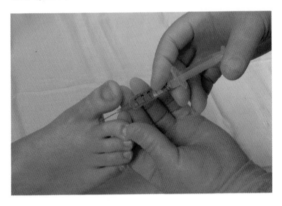

whilst injecting 3 ml of solution. Repeat in other
web spaces as appropriate.

Agent	Concn (%)	Volume (ml)	Onset (min)	Dur (h)
l-bupiv	0.5	3	20	6–12
lido	1	3	5–10	3–4

Web space block

This approach is in the horizontal plane (cf.
previous technique).
Surface landmarks Web spaces.
Patient position Patient supine with foot in
neutral position.
Technique Separate the toes of the required web
space as in Figure 2.33 and insert a 23G needle
into the web space in the horizontal plane to a

depth of 2 cm until the needle tip is level with the M-P joint. Inject 4 ml of solution. There should be no resistance to injection and the web space will distend slightly. Gentle massage of the distended space will disperse the solution around both dorsal and plantar digital nerves. In the conscious patient, web space block is the least uncomfortable technique if a 25G or 27G needle is used.

N.B. To avoid the risk of ischaemia, solutions containing vasoconstrictors should not be used.

High pressure within the confines of a web space, produced by excessive volume of injectate, must also be avoided. Limit volume to 4 ml of solution per web space.

Agent	Concn (%)	Volume (ml)	Onset (min)	Dur (h)
l-bupiv	0.5	4	30	6–12
lido	1	4	5	3–4

The abdomen and thorax

Introduction

For the surgery within the thorax and abdomen, central neural blockade using an epidural or a spinal technique is the only practical solution if regional anaesthesia is to be effective against both somatic and visceral pain. All painful stimuli arising from the visceral organs (including the pleura and peritoneum) are relayed via sympathetic visceral nociceptor nerve fibres to the spinal cord. Autonomic nerve blockade also offers other important benefits by preserving gut function, maintaining blood flow and modifying the neuro-humoral responses to surgical stress. Peripheral nerve blockade will not block viscerally mediated pain and cannot be used to provide adequate anaesthesia/analgesia for intra-abdominal surgery. The exception to the use of central neural blockade is the use of paravertebral blocks for unilateral surgery (breast, kidney and lung) because paravertebral blockade does produce segmental autonomic analgesia. For operations on the abdominal wall, which require mainly somatic analgesia, and where bilateral analgesia is unnecessary, peripheral nerve blocks are very effective at providing high quality postoperative analgesia. Even so, if abdominal contents are stimulated – if bowel is manipulated during herniorraphy for example – the patient may experience some visceral pain when undergoing hernia repair 'under local'.

Abdomen

Anatomy

Spinal nerves

The anterior abdominal wall is innervated by the 7th to the 12th thoracic nerves except in the inguinal area where the iliohypogastric and ilioinguinal nerves contribute to the somatic nerve supply. The nerves enter the abdominal wall through the transversus abdominis muscle and innervate the external and internal oblique muscles and the overlying skin before entering the posterior aspect of the rectus sheath. Here the nerves supply separate sections of the rectus muscles before leaving the anterior aspect of the sheath to innervate the midline skin of the abdomen. The subcostal nerve (T12) sends fibres

to the first lumbar nerve and its lateral cutaneous branch runs over the iliac crest to innervate the skin of the lateral aspect of the buttock as far as the greater trochanter.

Lumbar plexus

The majority of the lumbar plexus nerves innervate the lower limb (p 45). The nerve roots of L1 and 2, together with fibres from T12 supply the lowest cutaneous innervation of the abdominal wall, the suprapubic area and parts of the external genitalia. The fibres of T12 combine with L1 to form the iliohypogastric and ilioinguinal nerves (Figure 2.34), which sweep around the medial surface of the iliac crest and at a point 1–2 cm medial to the anterior superior iliac spine (ASIS) they are separated by the internal oblique muscle. The iliohypogastric nerve and the subcostal nerves lie between the internal oblique muscle and the aponeurosis of the external oblique while the ilioinguinal nerve lies deep to

Figure 2.34
Anatomy of the the iliohypogastric and ilioinguinal nerves

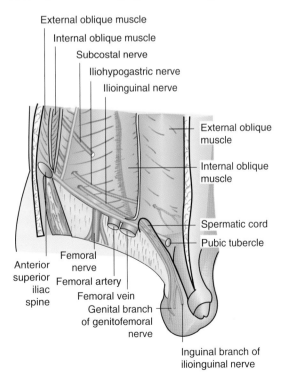

External oblique muscle
Internal oblique muscle
Subcostal nerve
Iliohypogastric nerve
Ilioinguinal nerve

External oblique muscle
Internal oblique muscle
Spermatic cord
Pubic tubercle

Anterior superior iliac spine
Femoral nerve
Femoral artery
Femoral vein
Genital branch of genitofemoral nerve
Inguinal branch of ilioinguinal nerve

Figure 2.35
Cutaneous innervation of iliohypogastric and ilioinguinal nerves

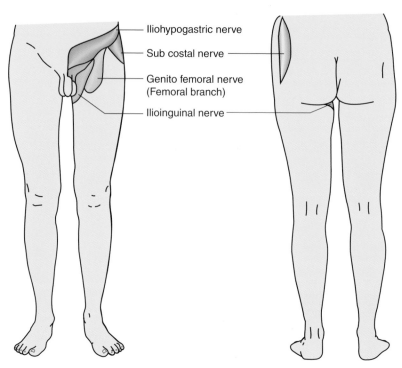

Iliohypogastric nerve

Sub costal nerve

Genito femoral nerve
(Femoral branch)

Ilioinguinal nerve

the internal oblique muscle. The iliohypogastric nerve innervates the skin overlying the lateral aspect of the buttock and then runs medially and superficial to the inguinal canal, to innervate the skin over the pubis. The ilioinguinal nerve enters the inguinal canal, accompanies the spermatic cord and supplies the skin of the root of the penis and anterior part of the scrotum (male) and the mons pubis and labium majorum (female). In addition, it innervates the skin of the upper and inner aspect of the thigh (Figure 2.35). The genitofemoral nerve (L1, 2) has two branches. The genital branch enters the inguinal canal and supplies the spermatic cord, innervating the same cutaneous area as the ilioinguinal nerve. The femoral branch innervates the skin overlying the femoral triangle.

Pudendal nerve

The pudendal nerve (S2, 3, 4) arises from the sacral plexus and gives rise to the dorsal nerve of penis (clitoris) and the perineal nerve. Each dorsal nerve passes under the pubic symphysis accompanied by the dorsal artery and vein running beneath the deep fascia of the penis into the

glans penis to supply the shaft and glans of the penis. Branches of the perineal nerve innervate the ventral surface and root of the penis. The perineal nerve also innervates the infero-posterior aspects of the scrotum (and labia majora in the female); Figure 2.36.

Applied anatomy

Any peripheral nerve block of the abdominal wall will only anaesthetise the somatic nerve supply to the abdomen. Such techniques are thus only suitable for operations which do not breach the peritoneum, although if the intra-abdominal component of the procedure is limited, there may be limited visceral pain and the somatic blockade will prove sufficient. Intercostal nerve blocks (p 78) are effective for unilateral analgesia of the anterior abdominal wall. The 7–11th intercostal nerves can be blocked by the standard approach to the intercostal space, but the 12th nerve can be difficult to locate under the 12th rib and therefore it is better to block this nerve more peripherally either by subcutaneous infiltration along the iliac crest (p 59) or by performing a discrete block of the

Figure 2.36
Innervation of (a) male and (b) female genitalia

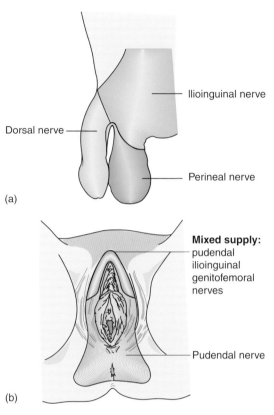

(a)

(b)

iliohypogastric nerve (p 77). Interpleural block provides the same distribution of analgesia as intercostal blocks but its effects will include somatic and autonomic blockade of the proximal thoracic spinal nerves and sympathetic chain. Paravertebral blocks produce extensive, unilateral, somatic and autonomic blockade of the thoracic and lumbar spinal nerve roots depending on the level at which they are blocked. Iliohypogastric and ilioinguinal nerve block is particularly indicated for surgery confined to the inguinal region and can be usefully combined with genitofemoral nerve block. This combination of nerve blocks is called the 'inguinal field block' to denote the area of analgesia produced.

Indications

Abdominal surgery

Intercostal blocks are well established in the management of post-operative pain from open cholecystectomy. Interpleural analgesia has been used for both laparoscopic and open cholecystectomy and nephrectomy but is not used as extensively as it once was, due to the reduction in the need for open cholecystectomy and the increasing use of paravertebral blocks.

Inguinal herniorraphy

The inguinal field block is suitable in both conscious and anaesthetised patients for hernia surgery and is especially useful in day surgery where it allows light general anaesthesia to be used, thus allowing a more rapid return to street fitness as well as offering prolonged post-operative analgesia.

Chronic pain conditions

Nerve entrapment syndromes occur in the abdominal wall, especially following surgery, and can be treated with appropriate paravertebral block, intercostal nerve block(s), rectus sheath block or inguinal canal block.

External genitalia
Anatomy

The external genitalia have a complex cutaneous nerve supply and it is therefore necessary to block several nerves if complete analgesia is to be achieved. This is impractical in females and a caudal epidural injection is more sensible. In the male, the penis, the scrotum and its contents can only be anaesthetised completely if the dorsal nerves of penis, perineal, genitofemoral and ilioinguinal nerves are all blocked.

Applied anatomy

Penile block (p 75) requires that the paired dorsal nerves of penis are blocked immediately beneath the deep ('Buck's') fascia at the inferior surface of the pubic symphysis to ensure that the posterior branches of the nerves, which innervate the ventral surface are affected, otherwise analgesia may be incomplete. Inguinal canal block (p 78) will block the ilioinguinal and genitofemoral nerves as well as the spermatic cord and the testicle and is therefore an essential technique to learn for testicular and scrotal surgery. Scrotal infiltration (p 76) along the line of anticipated incision is the most practical method of blocking the fibres of the pudendal nerves, which supply the scrotum.

Indications

Penile surgery

Penile blocks compare equally well with caudal blocks for circumcision and other penile surgery and avoid the inevitable side effects of caudals – bladder and bowel dysfunction and motor dysfunction in the legs. Depending on the type and site of surgery, a penile block may need to be combined with other blocks.

Scrotal/testicular surgery

Peripheral nerve blockade for testicular and scrotal surgery can be as effective as caudal or epidural techniques. For an inguinal approach to orchidopexy, an inguinal field block is the technique of choice but where testicular surgery is confined to the scrotum, an inguinal canal block with scrotal infiltration will be sufficient.

Thorax

For the majority of operations within the chest the regional anaesthetic technique of choice is central neural blockade using a thoracic epidural. Epidural analgesia is effective against both somatic and visceral pain and the autonomic nerve blockade offers important benefits by maintaining blood flow and modifying the neuro-humoral responses to surgical stress. Thoracic paravertebral blocks are increasingly popular for both intrathoracic and chest wall surgery. Single injections, either as a large bolus injected at a single level or small-volume injections repeated at multiple levels are used for breast and other chest wall procedures which require mainly somatic analgesia or where bilateral analgesia is inappropriate and unnecessary. Catheter insertion paravertebral techniques are indicated for intrathoracic procedures where prolonged post-operative analgesia is required.

Spinal nerves

The spinal cord gives rise to 12 pairs of thoracic nerves (T1–12), which share a number of common characteristics. All contain mixed motor, sensory and autonomic fibres and within the paravertebral space, divide into a small dorsal and larger ventral nerve. The dorsal nerves supply the erector spinae muscles and sensory fibres to the skin and deep structures of the posterior aspect

Figure 2.37
Dermatomes of the abdomen and thorax

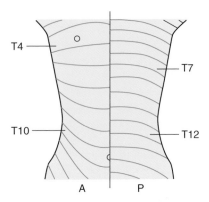

of the trunk. The ventral nerves supply the lateral and anterior parts of the trunk and each is contained within the neurovascular bundle of the intercostal space beneath the inferior aspect of the rib. Each nerve gives rise to a lateral branch and then continues forward to innervate the anterior aspect of the trunk. The sensory limits of each nerve are conventionally depicted as dermatomes on the skin surface (Figure 2.37), although there is considerable overlap between the individual dermatomes. T5, 7, 10 and 12 represent important landmarks on the trunk for the assessment of the spread of epidural or spinal analgesia.

As a result of the downward and forward paths of the thoracic nerves, posterior innervation stops at the level of the 12th thoracic spine. Anteriorly, the thoracic nerves supply the anterior abdominal wall and the subcostal nerve (T12) sends fibres to the first lumbar nerve and its lateral cutaneous branch runs over the iliac crest to innervate the skin of the lateral aspect of the buttock as far as the greater trochanter.

Applied anatomy

The number of nerves to be blocked will depend on the size and location of the injury or incision. It is necessary to block one nerve proximal and one distal to the selected nerve(s) because of the overlap of dermatomes. For example, a Kocher's subcostal incision for open cholecystectomy in the T7–8 dermatomes also requires T6 and 9 to be blocked for complete coverage.

For analgesia of the posterior part of the chest wall, a thoracic paravertebral injection (p 79), preferably with catheter insertion, is more suitable than intercostal nerve injections because the dorsal nerve is more reliably blocked and as the spread of a paravertebral injection is greater, fewer injections are required. Intercostal nerve blocks provide effective analgesia in the lateral and anterior parts of the chest wall. The technique is relatively easy to perform on the 6th to the 11th nerves as these ribs are easy to palpate but the scapula can obscure the higher ribs, thus the approach needs to be made more anteriorly which can reduce the effectiveness. Interpleural block is thought to achieve its effects by diffusion of local anaesthetic agent through the parietal layer of pleura causing blockade of the intercostal nerves, the sympathetic chain (and possibly the phrenic nerve). The block is not segmental and there may be little evidence of sensory anaesthesia. The spread of solution is greatly affected by gravity and the patient can thus be positioned so as to maximise the spread to the desired part of the pleural space. Tipping the patient head down in the supine position will block the upper thoracic nerves and the sympathetic chain and can induce Horner's syndrome.

Indications

Chest wall trauma

Fractured ribs can be treated by single injections around the appropriate intercostal nerves that may need to be repeated every 6–8 h.

Alternatively, catheters may be inserted into the intercostal spaces and a constant infusion of local anaesthetic solution or repeated bolus injections administered. Where there are multiple unilateral fractures, a paravertebral catheter is more appropriate because of the greater spread of solution. Thus a larger area of analgesia can be obtained from one catheter insertion and smaller volumes of local anaesthetic can be used. Alternatively, if the patient requires chest drains to be inserted, these can be used to produce interpleural analgesia.

Chest wall surgery

Interpleural blocks provide good analgesia for mastectomy or other breast operations. For thoracotomy incisions, a thoracic paravertebral injection offers better analgesia than intercostal blocks and because the chest is open, the surgeon can supervise the insertion of the catheter under direct vision. Thoracic paravertebral blocks are replacing interpleural blocks for breast surgery anaesthesia and are also used for post-operative

analgesia following renal surgery in preference to thoracic epidural infusions in some centres.

Chronic pain conditions

Nerve entrapment syndromes, thoracic spine pain and intercostal neuralgia may respond to paravertebral or intercostal blockade.

Bilateral or midline surgery or trauma

Bilateral intercostal, interpleural or paravertebral blocks should not be used because of the associated risks of drug toxicity and the need for multiple injection sites. A thoracic epidural is the technique of choice.

Peripheral nerve block techniques of the trunk

Abdomen

Penile block

Surface landmarks Symphysis pubis.
Patient position Supine.
Technique Stand on the right side of the patient. Palpate the distal edge of the symphysis pubis with the index finger of the left hand and introduce a 21G needle as in Figure 2.38, just distal to the index finger. Advance the needle until it contacts the distal leading edge of the pubis at which point it should have passed through the deep fascia of the penis ('Buck's' fascia). Inject 5–7 ml of solution after careful negative aspiration for blood. On no account should solutions contain any vasoconstrictor.

Provided that the needle is in the correct plane there is no need to re-position or make a second injection as both dorsal nerves are reliably blocked with this approach. Complete the block by making a subcutaneous injection of 3–5 ml of solution across the root of the penis. Start 2 cm lateral to the midline and inject continuously as the needle is advanced across the median raphe, finishing 2 cm beyond it on the other side (Figure 2.39). It is important to keep the needle subcutaneous in the midline because the urethra is very superficial at the base of the penis.

Agent	Concn (%)	Volume (ml)	Onset (min)	Dur (h)
l-bupiv	0.5	10	10	8

Figure 2.38
Penile block

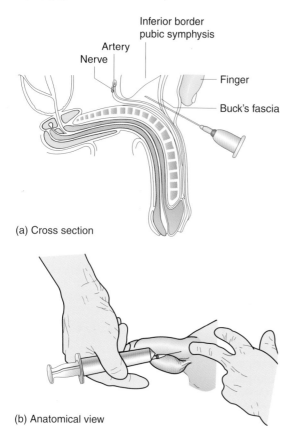

(a) Cross section

(b) Anatomical view

Figure 2.39
Penile block, completion

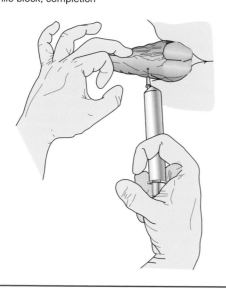

Figure 2.40
Scrotal infiltration

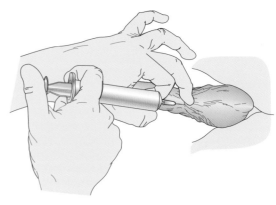

Scrotal infiltration

Unilateral or bilateral inguinal canal blocks need to be supplemented by scrotal infiltration to achieve complete analgesia of the testes (Figure 2.40). Make the injection in the median raphe if surgery involves both testes. For unilateral surgery, infiltrate over the anterior aspect of the relevant side of the scrotum. The injection should be made in consultation with the surgeon to ensure that it covers the site of the incision. If a vasoconstrictor is added to solution, it will aid haemostasis and indicate to the surgeon where to incise.

Agent	Concn (%)	Volume (ml)	Onset (min)	Dur (h)
l-bupiv + adren	0.5	10	5	8

Inguinal field block (Figure 2.41)

The technique requires discrete blockade of three nerves, the ilioinguinal, the iliohypogastric and the genitofemoral. In addition, subcutaneous infiltration of the abdominal wall is necessary to block overlapping nerve fibres from adjacent dermatomes.

Surface landmarks ASIS, pubic tubercle.
Patient position The patient is supine.
Technique Palpate the ASIS. Insert a 22G short bevel needle perpendicularly at a point 2 cm medial and inferior to the ASIS (a). Advance the needle carefully through the subcutaneous tissues until resistance indicates that the aponeurosis of the external oblique muscle has been reached. Move the needle from side to side,

Figure 2.41
Inguinal field block

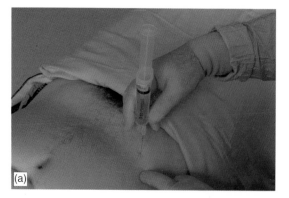

(a)

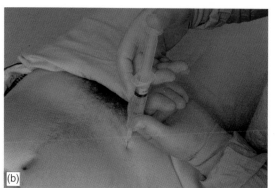

(b)

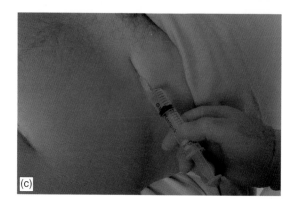

(c)

Figure 2.42
Infiltration at the lower end of the field block

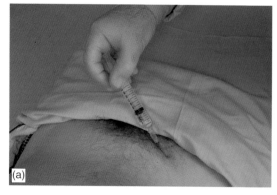

(a)

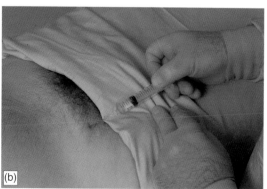

(b)

using two fingers of the other hand to move the skin over the underlying subcutaneous tissues. The needle will move easily and scratch on the aponeurosis. Advance the needle a little deeper and there will be a distinct 'pop' as it penetrates the tough fascia and side to side movement of the needle is no longer possible (b). The iliohypogastric nerve lies immediately deep to the aponeurosis and 5–7 ml of solution is sufficient to block it at this point. Now advance the needle a further 1–2 mm through the softer

resistance of the internal oblique muscle and inject a further 5–7 ml of solution to block the ilioinguinal nerve which is lying deep to the muscle before it penetrates the internal oblique to gain entry to the inguinal canal.

After the deep injection is complete, withdraw the needle to the skin and re-direct to inject a further 10 ml of solution subcutaneously in a fanwise distribution so that any cutaneous innervation from the subcostal nerve is blocked (c). An alternative technique involves a single injection of 15–20 ml just deep to the aponeurosis that should block both the iliohypogastric at the point of injection and the ilioinguinal distally as it emerges through the internal oblique muscle into the same plane as the iliohypogastric. The genito-femoral nerve is most reliably blocked by the inguinal canal block (p 78). If this is not possible due to an irreducible hernia or other anatomical abnormality, the lower end of the field block will require an injection of 10 ml of solution fanwise from the pubic tubercle towards the external inguinal ring and then towards the midline (Figure 2.42). This will block the fibres of genitofemoral and ilioinguinal as they emerge from the inguinal canal and also block any fibres, which cross the midline. Using up to 30 ml of concentrated local anaesthetic gives post-operative analgesia of 6–8 h. In the conscious patient it is necessary to use a larger volume of more dilute local because the surgeon may have to supplement the block with direct injection into some of the deeper structures.

Agent	Concn (%)	Volume (ml)	Onset (min)	Dur (h)
l-bupiv + adren	0.5	30	10	up to 8
l-bupiv + adren	0.25	40	20	3–4

Inguinal canal block

Inguinal canal block is indicated to supplement inguinal field block and also to anaesthetise the scrotal contents for a variety of urological operations. It is important to ensure that the inguinal canal contains only its normal structures (the spermatic cord and the ilioinguinal nerve) prior to performing this technique.
Surface landmarks ASIS, pubic tubercle and external inguinal ring.
Patient position Supine.
Technique Palpate the inguinal ligament between the ASIS and the pubic tubercle. Approximately 1 cm above its midpoint, the external inguinal ring can be palpated as a 'U'-shaped depression. In the obese patient or where previous surgery has made the landmarks difficult to palpate, the ring may be difficult to feel. In such cases, the skin of the scrotum can be invaginated with a finger and the external ring identified bimanually. Having confirmed that the inguinal canal contains no hernial contents, place the index finger (or the 5th finger) of the left hand on the deep ring to identify its position and insert a short bevel needle parallel to the inguinal ligament about 1 cm distal to the index finger, at 45° to the skin and aimed towards the external ring (Figure 2.43). There is usually a distinct 'pop' as the needle penetrates the external oblique aponeurosis and enters the inguinal canal. Hold the needle firmly in position, aspirate to ensure the needle is not intravascular and inject 5 ml of solution. The inguinal canal is usually 1–2 cm deep to the

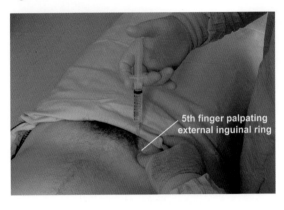

Figure 2.43
Inguinal canal block

5th finger palpating external inguinal ring

surface. It is important not to advance the needle too far once the canal has been entered because the femoral vessels and the femoral nerve lie immediately deep to the canal. If this block is used as part of an inguinal field block, after injecting 5 ml into the canal, the needle can be withdrawn to the skin and re-directed to inject a further 5–10 ml subcutaneously to complete the technique.

Agent	Concn (%)	Volume (ml)	Onset (min)	Dur (h)
l-bupiv	0.5	5	10	8

Thorax

Intercostal nerve block (Figures 2.45 and 2.46)

Surface landmarks Angle of each rib and mid-axillary line.
Patient position This will depend on whether the patient is anaesthetised or conscious. If anaesthetised or sedated, place the patient in lateral position, with side to be blocked uppermost. If conscious, sit upright on the edge of the bed, leaning forward onto a support.
Technique The anatomy of the intercostal space is shown in Figure 2.44. The ribs are easily palpated in patients of normal or thin build but in the obese patient they can be very difficult to define and this may be a relative contraindication to the technique. The same approach is used for each rib (Figures 2.45 and 2.46). Palpate the rib to identify the rib angle, which is usually found

Figure 2.44
Anatomy of the intercostal space

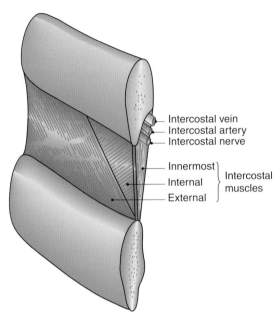

- Intercostal vein
- Intercostal artery
- Intercostal nerve

- Innermost ⎱
- Internal ⎬ Intercostal muscles
- External ⎰

8 cm lateral to the vertebral spine (Figure 2.45). The exact point of insertion of the needle is not crucial as long as it is posterior to the mid-axillary line, where the lateral cutaneous branch of the intercostal nerve arises. To identify the rib sequence, count the ribs upwards from the 12th rib, which is easy to identify due to its short length. Having reliably identified each rib, raise a skin bleb of local anaesthetic with a 25G gauge needle over each one and infiltrate down to the periosteum. Repeat for each intended level. Intercostal nerve blocks require multiple injections and many patients find them painful unless the anaesthetist is very gentle and sedation may be necessary. It may also be helpful to mark the sites of injection with a skin marker to lessen the likelihood of accidentally injecting the same space twice. Make the skin blebs at the inferior edge of the ribs so that when the main injection is made, the skin can be gently pulled cephalad with the index finger of the left hand until the point of insertion lies over the body of the rib (Figure 2.46a). Insert a 22G, 3 cm short bevel needle perpendicular to the skin until contact is made with the rib periosteum at which point support the needle firmly between thumb and index finger and 'walk' the needle off the inferior edge of the rib as the skin returns to its normal position (b). When the needle reaches the

inferior edge of the rib, cautiously advance 3–4 mm under the firm control of the left hand, braced against the patient's back (c). With short bevelled needles, a 'pop' may be felt as the needle penetrates the external intercostal muscle at its origin on the intercostal groove. Inject 3–4 ml of solution. As the thoracic nerves have both motor and sensory fibres, it is possible to use a nerve stimulator to identify each intercostal nerve by observing abdominal (not intercostal) muscle movement. In practice, however, nerve stimulators are rarely necessary for this procedure.

There is uncertainty about whether it is necessary to block each intercostal nerve to achieve a clinically effective block. Single space injections of a large volume have been described which may, in effect, replicate thoracic paravertebral injection. The intercostal space is a continuation of the paravertebral space and retrograde spread into the paravertebral space must be a possibility.

Pneumothorax is a major complication, the risk of which decreases with the experience of the practitioner. Nevertheless, the higher the number of spaces to be blocked, the greater the risk becomes. Any pneumothorax is usually minor but nitrous oxide administration may, however, increase the size of the gas volume.

Agent	Concn (%)	Volume (ml)	Onset (min)	Dur (h)
l-bupiv	0.5	3–4	10	4

Thoracic paravertebral block (Figure 2.47)

Surface landmarks Thoracic vertebral spinous processes.
Patient position Lateral with the injection side uppermost if anaesthetised. Sitting if conscious.
Technique Identify the spinous process of the appropriate thoracic vertebra, bearing in mind that because of the acute angulation of the thoracic spines the spinous process of the vertebra above the nerve to be blocked must be used. At a point 2.5–3 cm lateral to the cephalad edge of the spinous process, insert an 8 cm spinal needle at 90° to the skin and parallel to the midline (a) and advance until the contact with the

Figure 2.45
Intercostal nerve block position

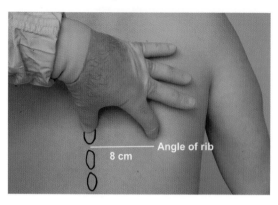

Figure 2.46
Intercostal nerve block

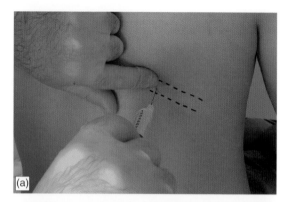

(a)

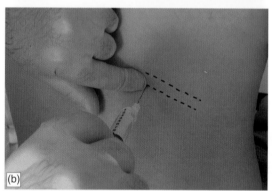

(b)

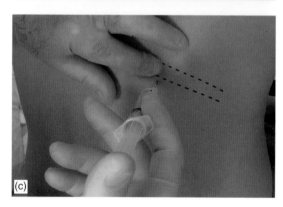

(c)

transverse process occurs, usually at a depth of 3–4 cm (b). Withdraw slightly, and re-angle cephalad so that the needle tip just 'walks off' the cephalad edge of the transverse process and advance a further 1–2 cm (c). It is important not to direct the needle medially as this may result in an epidural placement or inadvertent puncture of the dural cuff of the nerve. If the needle is directed laterally, it may produce an intercostal block or enter the pleural cavity. As the needle is advanced beyond the transverse process, it passes through the superior costotransverse ligament, often with a little 'click' or increase in tissue resistance depending on the state of ligament calcification to enter the paravertebral space. Loss of resistance to saline can be used to confirm the needle position (d) and in the conscious patient, paraesthesiae may occur in the distribution of the nerve. A peripheral nerve stimulator can also be used to confirm accurate needle placement, as pulse-synchronous movement of the rectus muscle should be visible. Careful aspiration to ensure that no cerebrospinal fluid (CSF) or blood is obtained should be followed by slow injection of the solution. The spread of local anaesthetic in the paravertebral space is very variable. As little as 5 ml may affect 1–6 dermatomes and can produce bilateral effects from penetration of the epidural space. On average, injecting 5 ml at one level blocks 3–4 dermatomes; if a more extensive spread is required, the procedure can be repeated at another space, or a catheter can be inserted (see p 128). Sequential doses may be given until the desired spread is achieved.

Complications: pneumothorax (up to 10% incidence), intrathecal injection and epidural spread.

Agent	Concn (%)	Volume (ml)	Onset (min)	Dur (h)
l-bupiv	0.5	5	10	4

Figure 2.47
Thoracic paravertebral block

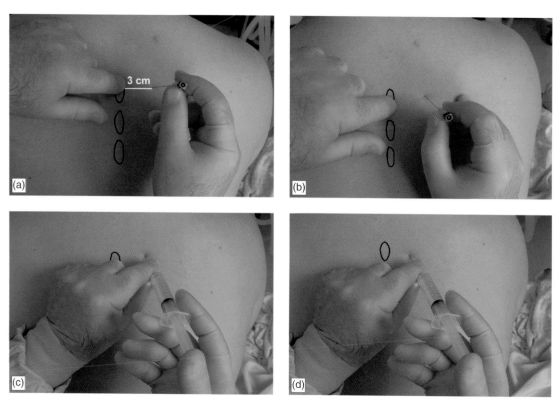

The upper extremity

Introduction

The brachial plexus provides most of the nerve supply to the upper limb, except for a small cutaneous area of the upper, medial aspect of the arm and the proximal part of the shoulder. These are innervated directly by nerve fibres from T2 and the superficial cervical plexus respectively. A single local anaesthetic injection around the brachial plexus therefore has the potential to provide surgical anaesthesia and prolonged post-operative analgesia to most of the upper limb. Five major terminal nerves to the limb arise from the plexus and these can be blocked singly or in combination to provide less extensive regional anaesthesia of the upper limb. The area of blockade can be extended or restricted according to the site of surgery and the degree of motor and sensory block required by performing nerve blocks at the level of the elbow or the wrist.

Brachial plexus

The brachial plexus is a complex neurological structure because the components of the plexus repeatedly combine and divide as they pass distally from the five cervical nerve roots to the level of the five terminal nerves within the axilla. For the purposes of regional anaesthesia, the configuration of the brachial plexus may be simplified by considering the major structural components and their relationships within the brachial plexus sheath (Figure 2.48). Furthermore, the brachial plexus, although complicated, has symmetry of structure, which helps to simplify the origins of the major components and clarify the ways in which it can be most effectively blocked (Figure 2.49).

Anatomy

The rule of 'fives and threes', applies to the structure of the brachial plexus (Figure 2.50).

Roots

The brachial plexus is formed from the ventral rami of C5–T1 with a variable contribution to the plexus from C4 (pre-fixed) and T2 (post-fixed). The roots emerge from the corresponding intervertebral foraminae of the cervical spine between the scalenus anterior and scalenus medius muscles within the posterior triangle of the neck. A fascial sheath, derived from the scalene muscles, invests the whole plexus as it passes laterally and distally over the first rib and beneath the midpoint of the clavicle to enter the axilla. The sheath can be detected as far distally as the midpoint of the humerus in some patients.

Trunks

The roots give rise to three trunks (superior, middle and inferior) arranged vertically over the first rib behind the midpoint of the clavicle.

Divisions

Each trunk divides into an anterior and posterior division behind the clavicle at the outer border of the first rib. The upper two anterior divisions join to form the lateral cord, the anterior division of the lower trunk continues singly as the medial cord and all three posterior divisions join to form the posterior cord.

Cords

The cords enter the axilla, arranged lateral, medial and posterior to the axillary artery, behind the pectoralis minor muscle. The lateral cord terminates as the musculocutaneous nerve and sends a root to form the median nerve. The medial cord sends an equivalent root to the median nerve and terminates as the ulnar nerve. The posterior cord terminates in two nerves – the axillary and radial.

Terminal nerves

The plexus gives rise to a total of 17 nerves, six supraclavicular and 11 infraclavicular. From a practical point of view only the suprascapular, ulnar, musculocutaneous, radial and median nerves can be blocked discretely. All the others will only be blocked as part of a brachial plexus block.

Figure 2.48
The brachial plexus

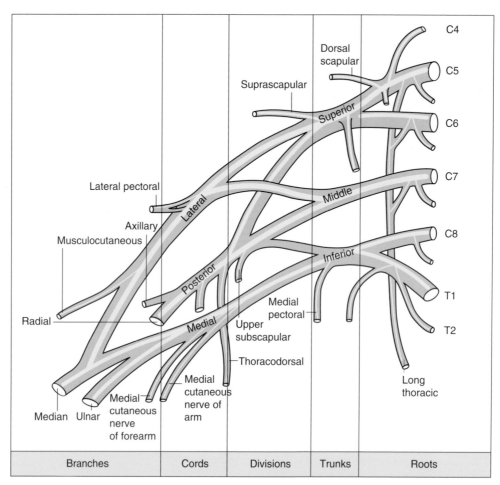

| Branches | Cords | Divisions | Trunks | Roots |

Figure 2.49
Nerves of the brachial plexus

Nerve	Main sensory branches
Axillary	Upper lateral cutaneous of arm
Radial	Lower lateral cutaneous of arm Posterior cutaneous of arm Posterior cutaneous of forearm Digital nerves of hand
Ulnar	Cutaneous to palm and dorsum of hand
Median	Cutaneous to palm and dorsum of hand
Musculocutaneous	Lateral cutaneous of forearm

Note: The medial cutaneous nerves of arm and forearm arise directly from the medial cord of the brachial plexus.

Figure 2.50
The rule of 'fives and threes', applying to the structure of the brachial plexus

Roots	5	C5–T1
Trunks	3	Superior (C5–6) Middle (C7) Inferior (C8–T1)
Divisions	3 3	Anterior Posterior
Cords	3	Lateral Medial Posterior
Nerves	5	Median (lateral and medial cords) Musculocutaneous (lateral cord) Ulnar (medial cord) Axillary (posterior cord) Radial (posterior cord)

Applied anatomy

The fascial sheath, which invests the brachial plexus from the scalene muscles down to the midpoint of the upper arm, is crucially important for successful brachial plexus blockade. At the proximal end of the plexus, the sheath usually offers obvious resistance to needle entry. More distally the sheath may contain internal septae, which can prevent uniform spread of local anaesthetic within the sheath and this has led to the development of multiple injection techniques. The two most important factors in determining the success of brachial plexus blockade are the volume of injectate and the level of entry into the sheath. In broad terms, the more distally the block is performed the larger the volume of local anaesthetic required. At the interscalene level, 20–25 ml will usually produce an effective proximal block. At the supraclavicular and infraclavicular levels 30–35 ml is necessary whilst in the axilla, up to 40 ml may be needed (all volumes quoted are for a fit 70 kg adult male).

The level of entry into the fascia will influence which components are preferentially blocked, and thus the resulting pattern of block. The interscalene approach is made at the level of the roots, usually close to C5 or 6. Therefore if there is incomplete blockade, C8 and T1 are most likely to be missed because of the vertical arrangement of the roots and the interscalene technique tends to fail on the ulnar side of the limb in a dermatomal distribution. The axillary approach is made at the level of the terminal nerves with inadequate block of the musculocutaneous and radial nerves being more likely because of the proximal origin of musculocutaneous and the posterior position of radial behind the humerus. Any failure of the block will be in a terminal nerve distribution. With the supraclavicular approach, injection is made at the level of the trunks. As there are only three components at this level, the failure rate should be low but if it does occur, it will be in a mixed distribution of terminal nerve and dermatomes derived from the inferior trunk. Similarly, the infraclavicular approach is made at the level of the three cords and any failure at this level will be a mixture of terminal nerve and dermatomes, possibly in the medial cord distribution.

The choice of approach depends primarily on the proposed site of surgery because the success rates of the different approaches vary.

The interscalene approach is best for proximal surgery on the shoulder joint and upper arm, the supraclavicular approach for the upper arm, elbow and radial side of forearm, and the infraclavicular and axillary approaches for the hand, wrist and forearm. To become proficient at all approaches requires considerable experience and for general use, confidence with one technique above the clavicle and one below is probably sufficient for most practitioners.

Indications

Shoulder surgery

An interscalene block is the plexus block of choice. If the incision is very proximal, separate superficial cervical plexus block (p 116) may be required. For closed procedures such as arthroscopy or manipulation, a suprascapular nerve block is often adequate.

Surgery of the upper arm and elbow

An interscalene or subclavian perivascular brachial plexus block is usually the best choice although the vertical infraclavicular approach can also be used. If the upper, medial aspect of the arm is involved, a separate intercostobrachial nerve block may be needed as well.

Forearm surgery

Depending on the extent and complexity of the operation, the vertical infraclavicular, axillary and subclavian perivascular approaches can all be used, with the exact site of surgery determining the best choice.

Wrist and hand surgery

An axillary or vertical infraclavicular block is indicated for major or prolonged surgery under tourniquet.

Trauma

Brachial plexus blockade provides rapid analgesia and anaesthesia for the reduction of joint dislocations of the shoulder and elbow and for the manipulation of fractures, where general anaesthesia may be contraindicated. Caution must be exercised with any form of regional anaesthesia used in forearm trauma where compartment syndrome may develop 'silently' with the dense analgesia masking the onset of pain. If the forearm needs extensive decompression and/or intercompartmental pressure monitoring is available then brachial plexus block may be used as indicated.

Chronic pain

The brachial plexus has a rich sympathetic nerve supply which controls both arterial and venous tone. Brachial plexus blocks can be used for diagnostic and therapeutic management of chronic pain conditions, many of which have a sympathetically maintained component. The dense somatic and sympathetic analgesia can be maintained for several days or even longer to enable prolonged rehabilitation of conditions such as complex regional pain syndrome. Ischaemic and vasospastic conditions also respond to prolonged blockade, as blood flow to compromised tissues following trauma and surgery will be maximised. The use of indwelling plexus catheters for prolonged brachial plexus analgesia is described in p 127.

Terminal nerves

All the motor and sensory nerves to the upper limb originate from the infraclavicular part of the brachial plexus but not all of them can be blocked discretely. The sensory and motor innervation of the upper arm and shoulder can only be blocked as part of a brachial plexus block. The terminal nerves to the forearm and hand can be blocked at the elbow (p 96) and the ulnar, median and radial nerves can also be blocked at the wrist (p 99).

Anatomy

Ulnar nerve

The ulnar nerve arises from the medial cord between the axillary artery and vein and passes down the medial aspect of the arm to enter the forearm, passing behind the medial epicondyle of the humerus. It supplies the flexor muscles of the forearm and passes down the ulnar side of the forearm. About 5 cm above the wrist, it gives rise to the dorsal and palmar cutaneous branches and then continues into the hand. The ulnar nerve is lateral and deep to the flexor

carpi ulnaris tendon, lying medial to the ulnar artery. The dorsal branch lies subcutaneously and dorsally at the level of the wrist joint and innervates the dorsal aspect of the little finger and the medial side of the ring finger. The palmar cutaneous branch supplies sensory innervation to the ulnar side of the palm. The deep branch supplies some of the intrinsic muscles and other deep structures plus palmar digital nerves to the little finger and the ulnar side of the ring finger.

Median nerve

The median nerve lies immediately medial to the brachial artery just proximal to the flexor skin crease of the antecubital fossa. At this point it is just deep to the bicipital aponeurosis in a groove bounded by the biceps tendon laterally and the origins of the forearm flexor muscles medially. It supplies the superficial and deep forearm flexors before it enters the hand deep to the flexor retinaculum in the carpal tunnel. The median nerve lies between the palmaris longus tendon medially and the flexor carpi radialis tendon laterally at a point about 2 cm proximal to the wrist. At this point, it gives off a superficial palmar cutaneous branch, which supplies the skin of the thenar eminence and the palm. The median nerve divides into its muscular branch (to the thenar muscles) and common digital branches distal to the flexor retinaculum and the latter divide at the level of the metacarpo-phalangeal joints to form the palmar digital nerves to the lateral three and a half digits (Figure 2.51).

Medial cutaneous nerve of the forearm

The medial cutaneous nerve of forearm lies subcutaneously above the bicipital aponeurosis in close relationship to the median nerve. It supplies the cutaneous innervation of the medial aspect of the forearm and some of the skin overlying the biceps in the upper arm.

Radial nerve

The radial nerve is the largest branch of the brachial plexus and passes posterior to the humerus through an intermuscular septum, then spirals round the humerus to supply the extensor muscles of the upper arm and the skin overlying them. It crosses the anterior

Figure 2.51
Innervation of the hand, (a) palmar and (b) dorsal view

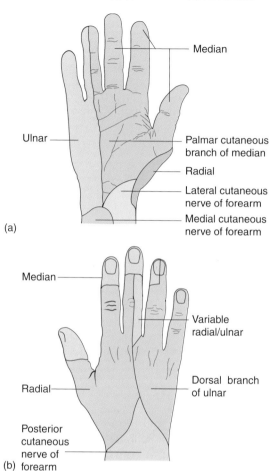

(a)

- Median
- Ulnar
- Palmar cutaneous branch of median
- Radial
- Lateral cutaneous nerve of forearm
- Medial cutaneous nerve of forearm

(b)

- Median
- Variable radial/ulnar
- Dorsal branch of ulnar
- Radial
- Posterior cutaneous nerve of forearm

aspect of the lateral epicondyle deep to brachioradialis to enter the forearm. The radial nerve emerges from deep to the tendon of brachioradialis and sends an interosseus branch to the back of the forearm to supply the supinators and extensors of the forearm and wrist. It then winds round the radius onto the dorsum of the wrist where it sends digital branches to the lateral three and a half digits.

Lateral cutaneous nerve of forearm

The lateral cutaneous nerve of forearm is the cutaneous continuation of the musculocutaneous nerve. It lies subcutaneously in the groove between brachioradialis and the biceps tendon and supplies the skin of the lateral aspect of the forearm.

Posterior cutaneous nerve of forearm

The posterior cutaneous nerve of forearm is a proximal branch of the radial nerve that becomes subcutaneous at the level of the elbow and descends along the postero-radial aspect of the forearm to innervate the overlying skin.

Digital nerves

The palmar aspect of each digit is supplied by two digital nerves, derived from either the ulnar nerve (5th finger and ulnar side of ring finger) or the median nerve (radial side of the ring finger, 2nd and 3rd fingers and thumb). These palmar digital nerves also innervate the dorsal aspect of the fingertips and nail beds.

The dorsal digital nerves are similar and derive from either the ulnar nerve (5th and ring finger) or the radial nerve (thumb and 2nd and 3rd fingers). They innervate the skin as far as the distal interphalangeal joint. There is considerable variation in the exact cutaneous territories supplied by each digital nerve especially at the boundaries of the three parent nerves.

Applied anatomy

The complex origins of the brachial plexus means that the cutaneous innervation of individual terminal nerves differs from the dermatomal pattern (Figure 2.52). The equivalent underlying myotomes and osteotomes of the muscles, bones and other deep structures do not correspond to the sensory distribution of skin overlying them. This means, for example, that blockade of the ulnar nerve will produce sensory loss on the ulnar side of the hand but motor loss in the flexor muscles of the forearm. These points are important when planning suitable techniques. It is usually necessary to block adjoining nerve territories for the majority of operations because there is considerable overlap and variation in the distribution of the peripheral nerves.

Elbow/forearm

The ulnar nerve runs in a narrow sulcus behind the medial epicondyle and should not be approached at this level because of the increased risk of damage either from the needle or from hydraulic pressure if excessive volume

Figure 2.52
Territories and dermatomes of the upper limb

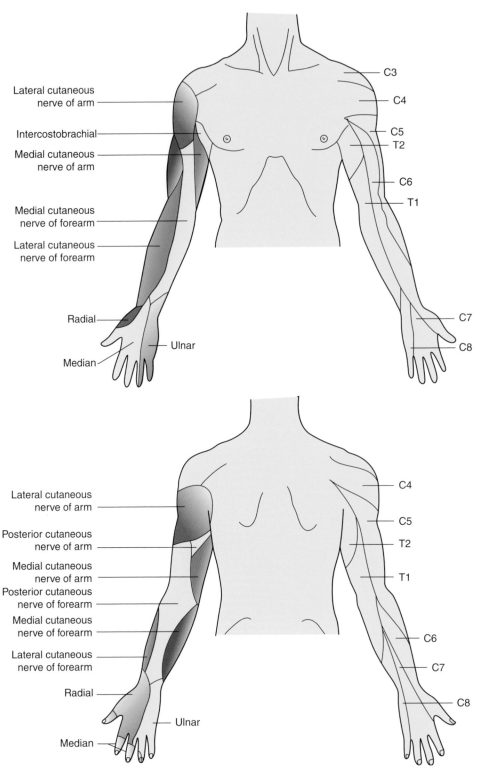

is injected into the confines of the sulcus. The median nerve is relatively superficial – often less than 1 cm deep to the skin. It is customary to block both the medial cutaneous nerve of forearm with the median nerve and the lateral cutaneous nerve of forearm with the radial nerve for complete forearm anaesthesia.

Hand

The terminal branches of the ulnar, median and radial nerves innervate the hand, with some overlap at the wrist of the medial, lateral and posterior cutaneous nerves of forearm. Although there is considerable overlap of the adjacent nerve territories in the hand, it is rarely necessary to block more than two nerves in combination unless the surgery is very extensive. In this case it is more sensible to use a more proximal technique such as a brachial plexus block.

If the proposed surgery involves a skin incision in the palm of the hand, the median nerve is better blocked at the elbow, as this will ensure that the palmar cutaneous branch is blocked. Otherwise the branch needs to be blocked separately at the wrist as part of the wrist block. Similarly, if the ulnar nerve is blocked at the wrist, the dorsal branch must be blocked separately. This is best done by the medial approach to the ulnar nerve rather than the ventral approach (p 99).

If surgery is limited to a single digit, then web space blocks are preferable to more proximal blocks because of the variable nerve supply. For surgery to multiple fingers the appropriate nerves should be blocked at the elbow or wrist as necessary.

Indications

Forearm surgery

The majority of operations on the upper limb are carried out distal to the elbow and this allows for the use of individual nerve blocks, either singly or in combination, to limit motor and sensory deficit to the nerve territories of the operative site. The combination of a short duration brachial plexus block and long-lasting peripheral nerve blocks is useful for day surgery as this combination allows early recovery of the shoulder and upper arm, important for early mobilisation and limb protection, while maintaining good peripheral analgesia.

Complex hand surgery

The nerves to the hand can be blocked either at the elbow or wrist according to the requirements of the operation. As with forearm surgery, if a tourniquet is necessary, brachial plexus anaesthesia may be the best option, unless general anaesthesia is used. Regional blocks at the wrist provide complete motor and sensory blockade of the hand whilst leaving the flexor and extensor muscles of the forearm unaffected. This can be of advantage in some forms of hand surgery where the patient remains able to move forearm muscles, to aid tendon identification.

Minor hand surgery

Nerve blocks at the wrist or digital nerve blocks are suitable for a variety of minor operations on the hand and fingers.

Post-operative analgesia

If a brachial plexus block is to be used for surgical anaesthesia, a short duration local anaesthetic can be used to produce rapid onset and recovery while individual nerves can be blocked distally with a long-acting local anaesthetic agent to provide prolonged analgesia in the hand. A combination of individual nerve blocks may be sufficient as the sole technique for less major surgery and they can be used to supplement general anaesthesia to provide prolonged post-operative analgesia.

Trauma

Minor trauma to digits can be managed with web space blocks or digital nerve blocks. If more than one digit is injured it may be more appropriate to consider discrete nerve blockade at the wrist. It is important to consider the risk of compartment syndrome occurring with closed injuries of the forearm unless the injury is to be decompressed.

Peripheral nerve blocks of the upper limb
Brachial plexus block

Brachial plexus block is probably the most frequently performed major peripheral nerve block. Since the earliest description of local infiltration of the cervical roots under direct vision by Halstead in 1885, over

40 techniques have been described in the literature. Many are slight modifications of the four major approaches, which can be categorised as interscalene, supraclavicular, axillary and infraclavicular. No one technique is ideal, as they have different benefits and complications and their use depends on which is most appropriate for the intended surgery. The interscalene approach is the best suited for shoulder and upper arm surgery but is difficult to learn and has the potential for very serious complications whereas the axillary approach is the easiest technique to learn, has the lowest incidence of complications but has relatively limited use except for hand surgery. The subclavian perivascular approach offers possibly the widest spectrum of spread from shoulder to hand but is associated with the risk of pneumothorax, limiting its popularity, especially in patients with respiratory disease. The vertical infraclavicular approach is the newest technique, first described in 1995. It is less uncomfortable and easier to perform than the original infraclavicular approach of Raj, it has a low profile of complications and has a high success rate.

With a fascial sheath investing the plexus, it is possible to influence the spread of solution by adjusting the volume of the injection to achieve the required area of anaesthesia for the proposed surgery. Winnie's monograph on brachial plexus blockade (1983), describes the relationships between the site of injection and the volume of injection and the use of digital pressure. The use of 40 ml of solution in a healthy male adult produced satisfactory spread whichever approach is used.

Patient positions for brachial plexus block are shown in Figure 2.53a–c.

Equipment

There are a number of needles designed for brachial plexus blockade, varying in length from 25 to 50 mm to suit the different approaches. Pencil point and short bevelled needles both increase the feedback from the fascia as the needle penetrates it, helping to improve placement accuracy and decrease the risk of nerve damage. By using a 10–20 cm extension tube, the needle can be isolated from the movements of the syringe during insertion, aspiration and injection or during changing of syringes – the 'immobile needle' concept. Peripheral nerve stimulators are now used

Figure 2.53
Patient positions for: (a) Axillary (b) interscalene and subclavian and (c) vertical infraclavicular

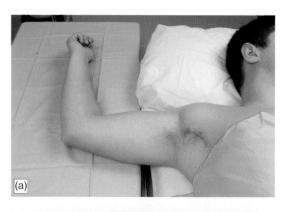

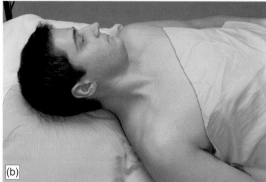

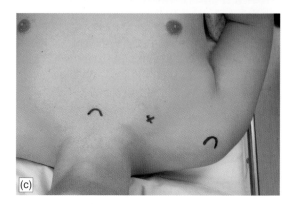

routinely to confirm accurate positioning of the needle for all approaches, although some experienced practitioners still perform axillary blocks successfully without the use of a PNS, using uninsulated needles.

Complications

Serious complications can occur with any of the approaches to the brachial plexus. Some

Figure 2.54
Complications of brachial plexus block

	Axillary	Supraclavicular	Interscalene	Comments
Vertebral artery injection	−	±	+ +	Rare but lethal
Subarachnoid/epidural injection	−	+	+ +	Rare but dangerous
Phrenic nerve palsy	±	+ +	+ + +	36–90% incidence usually asymptomatic
Recurrent laryngeal nerve palsy	−	+	+	1.5–6% incidence
Stellate ganglion block	+	+ +	+ + +	50–90% incidence
Pneumothorax	±	+ + +	+	0.6–25% incidence usually asymptomatic

complications are common to all regional anaesthetic techniques but others are specific to the different approaches (Figure 2.54).

Interscalene approach (Figure 2.55)

Landmarks Cricoid cartilage, posterior border sternomastoid muscle and interscalene groove.
Patient position Supine with a small pillow under the head and neck and the head turned slightly away from the side to be blocked. Push the shoulder downwards to depress the clavicle.
Technique Draw a line lateral from the cricoid cartilage to cross the sternomastoid at its midpoint. If the muscle is difficult to palpate, ask the patient to put it under tension by raising their head whilst keeping it turned to the side. Locate the interscalene groove behind the midpoint of the posterior border of the sternomastoid muscle with a palpating finger (a). Asking the patient to inspire vigorously or 'sniff' which will throw the anterior and middle scalene muscles into relief. Stand just behind the patient's head on the side to be blocked so that the needle insertion angle can be carefully controlled. Locate the interscalene groove and insert a 22G 25–35 mm short bevel needle at a point roughly level with the cricoid cartilage, aiming at an angle of 30° to the skin and slightly dorsal to the horizontal plane (b). This usually results in the needle being aligned with the nipple on the contralateral side in a definite caudad direction (c). It is very important that the needle is not aimed directly medial as described in some older interscalene techniques because this can increase the risk of the needle entering the intervertebral foramina and producing an epidural or intrathecal block, cervical nerve root or even spinal cord damage.

Figure 2.55
Brachial plexus block, interscalene approach

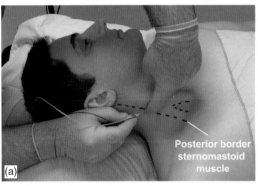

Posterior border sternomastoid muscle

(a)

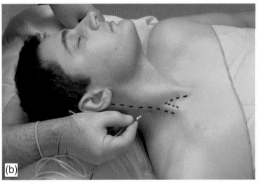

(b)

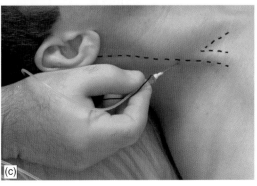

(c)

Some practitioners insert the needle higher up the interscalene groove with an angle to the skin of 20–30° aiming caudally to reduce further the risk of entering the intervertebral foramina. The fascial sheath will usually be entered with a 'pop' between 1 and 2 cm deep to the skin. Advance the needle slowly until paraesthesiae or pulse-synchronous muscle movements are elicited in the distribution of the arm or forearm (not the shoulder or neck). Aspirate to check for inadvertent entry into a vessel or a dural cuff, after which slow injection should be made with repeated aspiration.

Agent	Concn (%)	Volume (ml)	Onset (min)	Dur (h)
l-bupiv	0.5	20–25	30	8–12
ropiv	0.5	20–25	30	8–12
lido	1.5	20	20	4–6

Supraclavicular approach (subclavian perivascular technique) (Figure 2.56)

Landmarks Cricoid cartilage, posterior border of sternomastoid interscalene groove, clavicle and pulsation of subclavian artery.

Patient position Supine with a small pillow under the head and neck with the head turned slightly away from the side to be blocked.

Technique Stand just level with the top of the patient's head on the side of the neck to be blocked and gently push the shoulder downwards to depress the clavicle. Draw a line laterally from the cricoid cartilage to cross the sternomastoid at its midpoint (the external jugular vein often crosses the posterior border of the sternomastoid muscle at this point) (a). If the muscle is difficult to palpate, ask the patient to raise their head whilst keeping it turned to the side. The interscalene groove should be located behind the midpoint of the posterior border of the muscle. To highlight the groove, ask the patient to inspire vigorously or 'sniff' so that the middle and anterior interscalene muscles contract, emphasising the groove between them. Follow the interscalene groove down towards the clavicle. Approximately 1 cm above the midpoint of the clavicle, the pulsation of the subclavian artery can be felt in the interscalene groove. The ideal position for needle insertion is just above the

Figure 2.56
Brachial plexus block, supraclavicular block

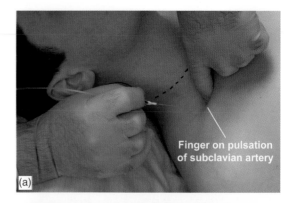

Finger on pulsation of subclavian artery

(a)

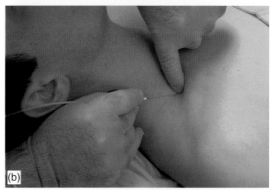

(b)

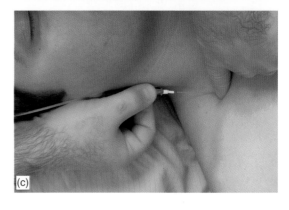

(c)

pulsation of the subclavian artery, although a more medial and proximal point is adequate as long as the groove is palpated with certainty (b). Insert a 22G short bevel 35 mm needle caudally in the horizontal plane, parallel to the midline (c). Marked resistance will give way to a 'pop' as the fascia is pierced 1–2 cm deep to the skin and paraesthesiae may occur. It is important to ascertain from the patient that the 'pins and needles' are in an appropriate distribution of the plexus (paraesthesiae around the shoulder should not be relied upon). Paraesthesiae most commonly occur in the distribution of the superior trunk because of the vertical arrangement of the nerve trunks. For the same reasons, a PNS will usually produce pulse-synchronous movement in the biceps or forearm extensors because of the C5/6 origins of the superior trunk. Once paraesthesiae or pulse-synchronous movement are elicited it is not necessary to hunt for other trunks. This will not increase the effectiveness of the block and just increases the risk of nerve damage or needle displacement from the sheath.

Hold the needle firmly in position and carefully aspirate to exclude intravascular placement, then inject slowly with frequent aspiration. If arterial blood is aspirated, carefully withdraw the needle until blood ceases to flow (because the subclavian artery is within the sheath, the needle will still be in the brachial plexus) and then inject. Solution should flow without resistance. Resistance or pain on injection may indicate intraneural injection and the needle must be re-positioned at once.

Up to 40 ml of solution can be used depending on the mass of the patient and the sheath may be felt to distend during the injection; this is normal and is easily distinguished from the subcutaneous swelling of an extra-fascial injection.

Agent	Concn (%)	Volume (ml)	Onset (min)	Dur (h)
l-bupiv	0.5	25–40	30	8–12
ropiv	0.5	25–40	30	8–12
lido	1.5	25–40	20	3–5

Axillary approach (Figure 2.57)

Landmarks Axillary artery pulsation and lateral border of pectoralis major.
Position Supine with the arm abducted to 90° at the shoulder and the elbow flexed to 90° (Figure 2.57). Do not over-abduct the arm because the pulsation of the artery may be diminished by pressure from the head of the humerus.
Technique Palpate the pulse of the axillary artery level with the lateral border of the pectoralis major and fix the artery with the palpating finger (a). Insert a 35 mm 22G short bevel needle just superior to the artery until the

Figure 2.57
Axillary block

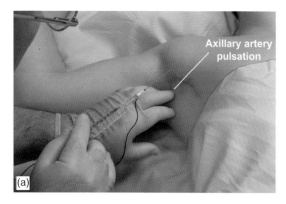

Axillary artery pulsation

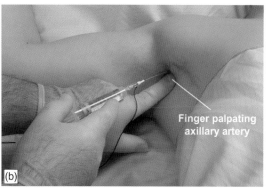

Finger palpating axillary artery

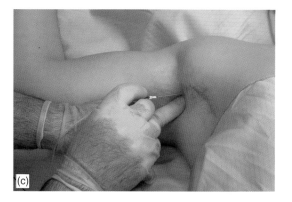

resistance of the fascial sheath is felt and a 'pop' indicates that the needle has entered the sheath (b). Paraesthesiae indicate correct needle placement and a PNS can be used to confirm this. After negative aspiration, inject the local anaesthetic solution (c) and after the injection is complete, adduct the arm so that the humeral head no longer obstructs the proximal spread of solution. If blood is aspirated at any stage of the injection, this indicates intra-arterial needle placement and in this case the needle can either be withdrawn and re-positioned within the sheath or it may be deliberately advanced further until no more blood can be aspirated and the injection made deep to the artery (the transarterial technique).

The *musculocutaneous nerve* may not be blocked adequately by the axillary approach and can be blocked separately after completion of the axillary injection by withdrawing the needle from the sheath and re-directing it at 90° to the skin and superior to the artery. Advance the needle into the coracobrachialis muscle and inject 5–7 ml of solution. The usual reason to block the musculocutaneous nerve is to improve sensory block in the territory of its cutaneous distribution – the lateral cutaneous nerve of forearm and this can be done very easily at the elbow instead (p 98).

The *intercostobrachial nerve* is not part of the brachial plexus and may need to be blocked separately in the axilla to provide analgesia to the upper, inner aspect of the arm. From the same needle insertion point as for the axillary approach to the brachial plexus, withdraw the needle to the subcutaneous tissues, angle medially and inject 3–5 ml of solution.

Agent	Concn (%)	Volume (ml)	Onset (min)	Dur (h)
l-bupiv	0.5	30	25–35	12
ropiv	0.75	40	25–35	12

The vertical infraclavicular block

Landmarks Sternoclavicular joint (SCJ), midpoint of the clavicle (MP) and ventral aspect of the acromion (Ac).
Position Supine with the head on a small pillow.
Technique The key to success is accurate marking of the landmarks. Use a skin marker to locate the sternoclavicular joint and the ventral tip of the acromion. To locate the latter accurately, palpate the lateral end of the clavicle and then the acromioclavicular joint, moving the finger ventrally (anteriorly) to the tip of the acromion. Move the arm passively and with the finger in the correct place you should be able to feel the head of the humerus moving distal to the fixed tip of the acromion. Measure the distance between the two landmarks (usually about 18–19 cm in an adult male) and mark the

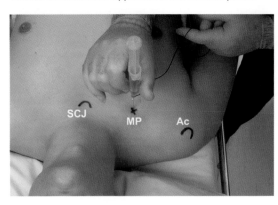

Figure 2.58
Vertical infraclavicular approach to the brachial plexus

halfway point immediately below the clavicle (Figure 2.58). Insert a 50 mm short bevelled insulated needle in the strictly vertical plane, checking continuously that the needle is vertical to the skin in all planes. Deep to the subcutaneous tissue the pectoral muscles offer a slight resistance to needle insertion and will produce muscle movement when the PNS is turned on. Between 2 and 4 cm the needle should contact one of the brachial plexus cords around the axillary artery – usually the lateral cord, producing movements in the distribution of the musculocutaneous and median nerves. Less frequently, if the needle is inserted more medially, the medial cord may be stimulated, producing movements in the distribution of the ulna nerve. Do not insert the needle deeper than 4 cm as the risk of pneumothorax increases beyond this depth. Once pulse-synchronous movement is elicited, aspirate and then slowly inject up to 40 ml of local anaesthetic.

Agent	Concn (%)	Volume (ml)	Onset (min)	Dur (h)
l-bupiv	0.5	30	25–35	12
ropiv	0.75	40	25–35	12

Suprascapular nerve block

Posterior approach

Landmarks Spine of scapula.
Position Sitting position.
Technique Palpate the length of the spine of the scapula and identify its midpoint – the

Figure 2.59
Suprascapular nerve block, posterior approach

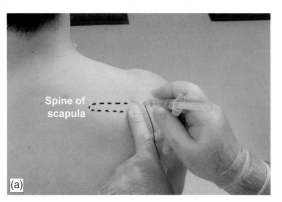

(a)

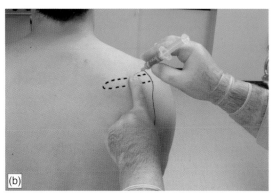

(b)

Figure 2.60
Suprascapular nerve block, superior approach

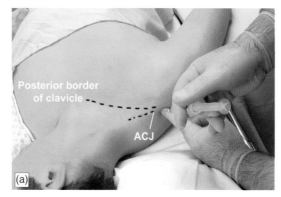

(a)

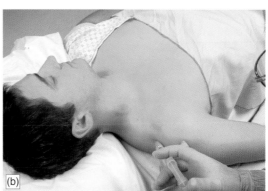

(b)

suprascapular notch is approximately 1 cm above it. Insert a 22G short bevel needle at right angles to the skin to a depth of 2–3 cm at which point bony contact will usually occur (Figure 2.59). Carefully move the needle to locate the edges of the suprascapular notch at which point it will produce paraesthesia in the shoulder if the nerve is contacted (or a PNS can be used to locate it). It is important not to insert the needle into the notch to avoid nerve damage and the needle must not be angled superiorly in case it passes anterior to the scapula.

Agent	Concn (%)	Volume (ml)	Onset (min)	Dur (h)
l-bupiv	0.5	5–7	15	8–12
ropiv	0.75	5–7	10	8–12

Superior approach

Landmarks The posterior border of clavicle and the acromioclavicular joint (ACJ).

Position Supine.
Technique Locate the medial aspect of the acromioclavicular joint by palpating the posterior border of the clavicle until no more lateral progress can be made (Figure 2.60). The trapezius muscle may cover the joint at this point but the joint should be palpable beneath the muscle. At this point insert a 70 mm insulated 22G short bevel needle aiming slightly dorsally (posteriorly) and towards the contralateral nipple. At a depth of about 3 cm connect a nerve stimulator and advance the needle tip until pulse-synchronous contraction of supraspinatus occurs, initiating abduction of the shoulder If the needle is inserted too deeply bone will be felt as the needle impinges on the medial border of the suprascapular notch or the spine of scapula. With correct needle placement, injection of 5–6 ml of local anaesthetic will produce instant fade of the PNS movement of the shoulder and this should reduce any confusion with unwanted direct stimulation of trapezius, which may be seen if the needle is too superficial.

Agent	Concn (%)	Volume (ml)	Onset (min)	Dur (h)
l-bupiv	0.5	5–7	15	6–12
ropiv	0.75	5–7	10	6–12

Figure 2.61
Ulnar nerve block

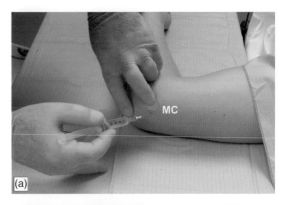

(a)

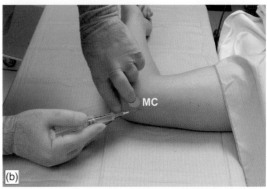

(b)

Nerve blockade at the elbow

The ulnar, median and radial nerves may be approached singly or in combination at the elbow to provide sensory loss to the hand and motor loss to the forearm muscles and the intrinsic muscles of the hand. If sensory loss to the forearm is required, then the lateral, medial and posterior cutaneous nerves of the forearm must be blocked separately at the elbow. Any of these nerves can also be blocked to reinforce a brachial plexus block is that would otherwise be inadequate for surgery.

Ulnar nerve block (Figure 2.61)

Landmarks Medial epicondyle of humerus (MC) and ulnar sulcus.
Position Abduct the arm to 90° at the shoulder, supinate the forearm and flex the elbow to 90° (a).
Technique Palpate the medial epicondyle of the humerus. It is often possible to 'roll' the nerve beneath the palpating finger just proximal to the epicondyle before the nerve enters the sulcus behind the condyle. Insert a 25 mm 22G short bevel needle 1–2 cm. proximal to the epicondyle in the horizontal plane (b) and gently advance until paraesthesiae are elicited or until the needle strikes bone in which case, withdraw slightly and re-position. The nerve is superficial and the needle rarely needs to be inserted more than 0.5–1.0 cm. Inject 3–4 ml of solution slowly. The injection should be of low resistance and cause no pain or paraesthesiae. Resistance to injection or pain indicates intraneural injection and the injection should be stopped immediately and the needle re-positioned. If the nerve is difficult to locate, a PNS may be used to confirm its position when pulse-synchronous flexion of fingers and wrist will be seen.

To avoid the possibility of nerve damage, do not inject within the sulcus of the medial epicondyle. At this point, the nerve is tightly restricted by the medial ligament of the

elbow and thus cannot move away from the advancing needle tip. It may also be exposed to high-pressure ischaemic damage if a large volume of solution is injected into this small channel.

Agent	Concn (%)	Volume (ml)	Onset (min)	Dur (h)
l-bupiv	0.5	4	15	12
ropiv	0.5	4	10	8–10
lido	1	5	10	4

Median nerve block (Figure 2.62)

Landmarks Antecubital fossa, brachial artery pulse, medial border of biceps tendon and humeral head of pronator teres.
Position Abduct the arm at an angle of 45°, in supine extension (a).
Technique Identify the pulse of the brachial artery in the intermuscular groove between the biceps tendon and the head of pronator teres, just proximal to the flexor crease of the

Figure 2.62
Median nerve block

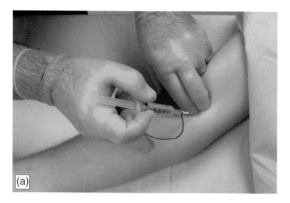

(a)

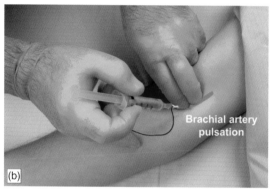

(b)

Brachial artery pulsation

antecubital fossa. Insert a 25 mm 22G short bevel needle at an angle of 45° to the skin just medial to the brachial artery and 1–2 cm proximal to the flexor skin crease of the antecubital fossa (b). There may be a 'pop' or loss of resistance as the needle penetrates the bicipital aponeurosis beneath which the nerve lies. If paraesthesiae are produced, aspirate and inject 4–5 ml of solution slowly. A PNS may be used and will stimulate pulse-synchronous flexion of fingers and wrist.

Agent	Concn (%)	Volume (ml)	Onset (min)	Dur (h)
l-bupiv	0.5	5	15	12
ropiv	0.75	5	10	8–10
lido	1	5	10	4

Medial cutaneous nerve of forearm block

Landmarks See median nerve block.
The medial cutaneous nerve of the forearm is usually blocked in conjunction with the

Figure 2.63
Medial cutaneous nerve of forearm, anterior view

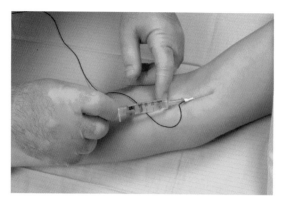

median nerve and requires the same landmarks. On completion of the median nerve block, withdraw the needle to the subcutaneous tissue and then advance proximally along the intermuscular groove whilst injecting a 'sausage' of up to 7 ml of solution (Figure 2.63).

Agent	Concn (%)	Volume (ml)	Onset (min)	Dur (h)
l-bupiv	0.5	5–7	15	12
ropiv	0.75	5–7	10	8–10
lido	1	5–7	10	3–4

Radial nerve block (Figure 2.64)

Landmarks Antecubital fossa (acf), lateral epicondyle of humerus, lateral border of biceps tendon (BT) and medial border of brachioradialis muscle (BM).
Position Arm abducted to 45° in supine extension.
Technique Identify the intermuscular groove between the biceps and brachioradialis just proximal to the flexor skin crease of the antecubital fossa (a). The nerve runs deep to the brachioradialis muscle at this point and can be difficult to locate without using a PNS (motor response will be extension of fingers and wrist and abduction of thumb). Identify the lateral epicondyle and place a finger underneath it to act as a guide for the direction of needle insertion (b). Insert a 35 mm 22G short bevel needle into the intermuscular groove approximately 2 cm proximal to the flexor skin crease of the antecubital fossa and aim towards the lateral epicondyle. Paraesthesiae (or pulse-synchronous movement in the

Figure 2.64
Radial nerve block

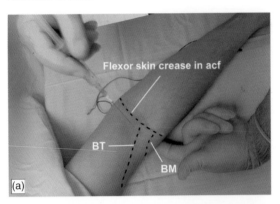

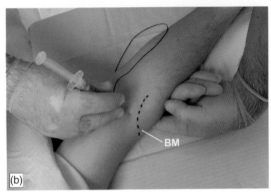

Figure 2.65
Lateral cutaneous nerve of the forearm block

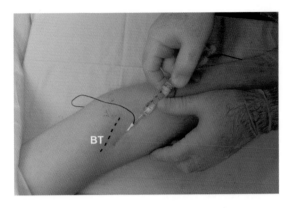

Figure 2.66
Posterior cutaneous nerve of the forearm block

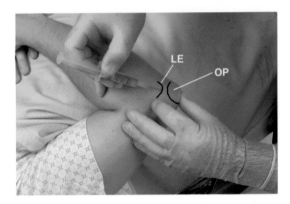

distribution of the nerve) may occur before the needle strikes bone in which case 5–7 ml of solution should be injected. Otherwise the needle must be re-directed more medially until the nerve is found.

to lie parallel with the tendon and inject 5–7 ml of solution (Figure 2.65).

Agent	Concn (%)	Volume (ml)	Onset (min)	Dur (h)
l-bupiv	0.5	7	15	12
ropiv	0.75	5–7	10	8–10
lido	1	10	10	4

Agent	Concn (%)	Volume (ml)	Onset (min)	Dur (h)
l-bupiv	0.5	5–7	15	12
ropiv	0.75	5–7	15	8–10
lido	1	5–7	10	4

Lateral cutaneous nerve of forearm block

Landmarks See radial nerve block.
The lateral cutaneous nerve of forearm is usually blocked in conjunction with the radial nerve and the same landmarks are required. After completion of the radial nerve block, withdraw the needle so that it is just deep to the deep fascia and lateral to the biceps tendon in the intermuscular groove. Re-direct the needle

Posterior cutaneous nerve of forearm block

Landmarks Lateral epicondyle (LE) of humerus and olecranon process (OP).
Position Flex the arm across the chest of the patient.
Technique From a point directly over the lateral epicondyle, inject a subcutaneous 'sausage' of solution medially between the two landmarks (Figure 2.66).

Agent	Concn (%)	Volume (ml)	Onset (min)	Dur (h)
l-bupiv	0.5	5	15	12
ropiv	0.75	5	15	8–10
lido	1	5	10	4

Hand and wrist

Nerve blockade at the wrist will produce sensory loss of the hand and motor loss of the intrinsic muscles of the hand (but not of the extensors and flexors of the hand and wrist).

Ulnar nerve block

There are two methods of approaching the nerve, ventral and medial. The medial approach reduces the risk of ulnar artery damage because the artery is lateral to the nerve. The medial approach is also preferable because both the dorsal and palmar cutaneous branches may be blocked from the same needle insertion point.

The ventral approach (Figure 2.67)

Landmarks Flexor carpi ulnaris tendon (FT), ulnar artery pulse and pisiform bone.
Position Place the arm in supine extension supported on a small sandbag above the wrist.
Technique Identify the flexor carpi ulnar tendon approximately 1 cm proximal to its insertion into the pisiform at the skin crease of the wrist (a). It is usually possible to palpate the ulnar artery at this point and the ulnar nerve lies medial to the artery and deep to the radial border of the tendon. Advance a 25G gauge needle perpendicular to the skin between the flexor carpi ulnaris tendon and the ulnar artery pulsation (b) until paraesthesiae are elicited approximately 1 cm deep to the skin. Slowly inject 3–4 ml of solution and then withdraw the needle to the subcutaneous tissue where a further 2–3 ml should be injected to block the palmar cutaneous branch.

Agent	Concn (%)	Volume (ml)	Onset (min)	Dur (h)
l-bupiv	0.25	7	10	6–12
lido	1	7	10	4

Medial approach (Figure 2.68)

Landmarks Flexor carpi ulnaris tendon, ulnar artery pulse and pisiform bone.

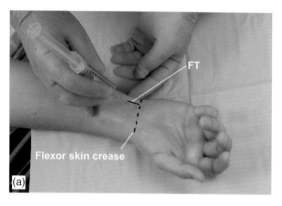

Figure 2.67
Ulnar nerve block, ventral approach

FT
Flexor skin crease
(a)

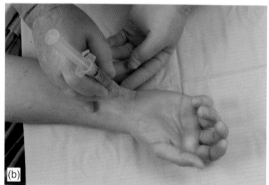

(b)

Position The arm in supine extension and supported on a small sandbag above the wrist.
Technique Insert a 25G needle at 90° to the skin immediately deep to the flexor carpi ulnaris tendon about 1 cm proximal to the pisiform bone (a). At a depth of 1–1.5 cm, slowly inject 3–4 ml of solution and withdraw the needle to the subcutaneous tissue where it should then be re-directed both dorsally to block the dorsal branch with 2 ml of solution and ventrally to block the palmar branch with 2 ml of solution (b).

Agent	Concn (%)	Volume (ml)	Onset (min)	Dur (h)
l-bupiv	0.25	6	20	6–12
lido	1	6	5	3–4

Median nerve block (Figure 2.69)

Landmarks Flexor carpi radialis tendon and palmaris longus tendon (if present) (PLT).

Figure 2.68
Ulnar nerve block, medial approach

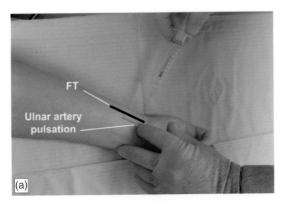

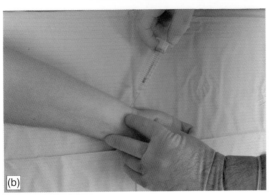

Figure 2.69
Median nerve block

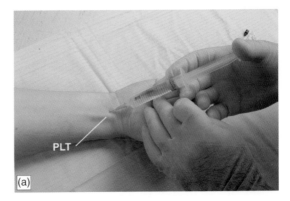

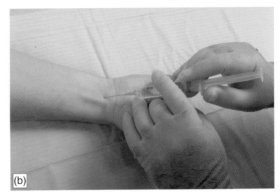

Position Place the arm in supine extension, supported on a small sandbag above the wrist.
Technique Ask the patient to flex the wrist against resistance and, if present, the tendon of palmaris longus will be highlighted. Insert a 25G needle just lateral to the tendon. In the absence of palmaris longus, insert the needle 1 cm medial to the ulnar border of flexor carpi radialis tendon (a). At a depth of up to 1 cm, increased resistance indicates that the flexor retinaculum has been reached and the needle should be slowly advanced a further 2–3 mm. The nerve lies immediately deep to the retinaculum and as soon as paraesthesiae are elicited, immobilise the needle and carefully inject 3–4 ml of solution. Resistance to injection or pain may indicate intraneural injection in which case, withdraw and re-position the needle. On completion of the median nerve block, withdraw the needle to the subcutaneous tissue and inject a further 2 ml of solution to block the palmar cutaneous branch (b). Do not use this approach in the presence of carpal tunnel syndrome due to the tight restriction of the nerve beneath the retinaculum.

Agent	Concn (%)	Volume (ml)	Onset (min)	Dur (h)
l-bupiv	0.25	6	20	6
lido	1	10	5	2

Radial nerve block

Landmarks Styloid process of ulna, styloid process of radius, tendon of extensor pollicis brevis and tendon of extensor pollicis longus.
Position Place the arm in prone extension, abducted from the body.
Technique If the thumb is extended against resistance, the tendons will be thrown into relief and the 'anatomical snuff box' can be identified, overlying the styloid process of the radius. At this level, the radial nerve is subcutaneous and has already divided into its terminal branches to the thumb and radial aspect of the dorsum of the hand. Insert a 22G 3.5 cm needle close to the tendon of extensor pollicis longus over the styloid process of the radius and direct it subcutaneously across the dorsum of the wrist towards the ulnar border of the wrist along a

Figure 2.70
Radial nerve block

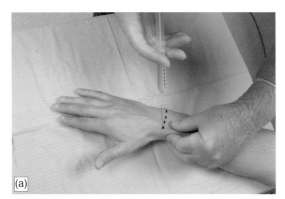

(a)

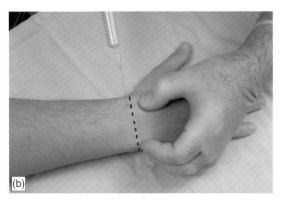

(b)

Figure 2.71
Digital nerve block, metacarpal approach

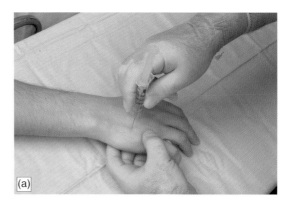

(a)

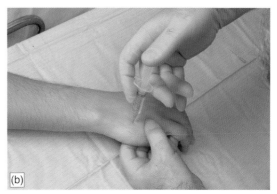

(b)

line joining both styloid processes. Inject a 5–7 ml 'sausage' of solution as the needle is advanced (Figure 2.70b). Withdraw the needle to the insertion point and re-direct it across the tendon of flexor pollicis brevis and inject a further 2–3 ml of solution subcutaneously (Figure 2.70a). This technique may more properly be considered a field block rather than a discrete nerve block.

Agent	Concn (%)	Volume (ml)	Onset (min)	Dur (h)
l-bupiv	0.5	10	30	12
ropiv	0.75	10	20	8–10
lido	1	10	15	4

Digital nerve block

There are three approaches to the digital nerves of the hand: metacarpal, classical and web space. The metacarpal approach is perhaps more painful for the patient and should be reserved for those occasions when anaesthesia of the intrinsic muscles and other deep structures of the hand is required. When anaesthesia of the fingers alone is required, both the classical dorsal approach to the digital nerves and the web space approach are equally satisfactory, although the latter is more comfortable for the conscious patient.

Metacarpal block

Landmarks Inter-metacarpal spaces.
Position The hand should be prone.
Technique Identify the inter-metacarpal spaces corresponding to the fingers to be blocked at their midpoints. Insert a 25G needle perpendicular to the skin and direct it vertically towards the palmar surface of the hand (Figure 2.71). Place a finger on the palm beneath the space to detect the needle as it approaches the palmar aponeurosis. Do not pierce the aponeurosis because the digital nerves lie deep to the aponeurosis. Inject 2 ml of solution at the aponeurosis, a further 2 ml as the needle is withdrawn and then a final 2 ml at the level of the dorsal border of the metacarpal.

Figure 2.72
Digital nerve block, perpendicular approach

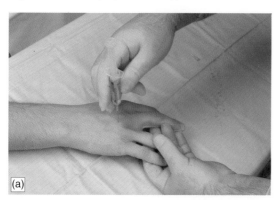

(a)

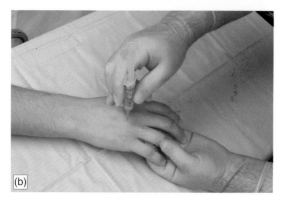

(b)

Figure 2.73
Web space block

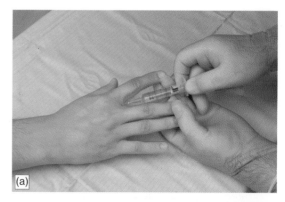

(a)

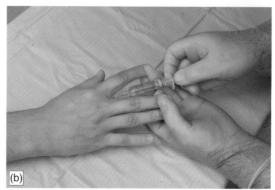

(b)

Agent	Concn (%)	Volume (ml)	Onset (min)	Dur (h)
l-bupiv	0.5	6	20	12
lido	1	6	20	4

Digital nerve block – perpendicular

Landmarks Metacarpo-phalangeal joints and web spaces.
Position The hand should be prone.
Technique Identify the appropriate metacarpo-phalangeal joints and insert a 25G needle perpendicular to the skin, just distal to the joint. Place a finger on the palmar surface to detect the needle as it advances towards the palmar border of the phalanx (Figure 2.72). With the needle at its deepest position slowly inject 3 ml of solution as the needle is withdrawn.

Agent	Concn (%)	Volume (ml)	Onset (min)	Dur (h)
l-bupiv	0.5	3	20	12

Web space block

Landmarks Web spaces.
Position Place the hand prone with the fingers separated.
Technique Approach the digital nerves in the horizontal plane by separating the fingers that delimit the space and insert a 25G needle into the web space to a depth of 2 cm until the needle tip is level with the metacarpo-phalangeal joint (Figure 2.73). After negative aspiration, inject 5 ml of solution. There should be no resistance to injection but the web space will distend slightly. Gently massage the space to disperse the solution around the dorsal and ventral nerves after removing the needle. To avoid causing ischaemia to the digits, do not use local anaesthetic solutions that contain vasoconstrictors. Hydraulic pressure ischaemia due to large-volume injection should be avoided by limiting the volume to 5 ml per space or less.

Agent	Concn (%)	Volume (ml)	Onset (min)	Dur (h)
l-bupiv	0.5	5	20	12

Ophthalmic surgery (Monica Hardwick)

Introduction

The majority of operations within the orbit can be accomplished under regional anaesthesia and cataract surgery is routinely carried out under regional anaesthesia in day-stay surgical units in many centres. Either the surgeon or anaesthetist may perform the regional anaesthesia for ophthalmic surgery, provided that they receive appropriate training in performing the techniques, are fully conversant with the associated risks and complications and can treat them accordingly.

Anatomy

Orbit

The orbit contains the eyeball (globe), the extra-ocular muscles, the lacrimal gland and the associated nerve and blood supplies. The surrounding structures of the orbital margins are supplied by vessels and nerves that traverse the orbit.

Extra-ocular muscles

There are seven extra-ocular muscles in total; one controls the upper eyelid (levator palpebrae superioris) and the other six control movement of the globe. The four rectus muscles (superior, inferior, medial and lateral) arise from a common tendon around the optic foramen and form an incomplete cone of muscle as they pass forward to their insertions on the globe. Within the cone are: the ophthalmic artery, the ciliary ganglion and the optic cranial nerve (CN II), oculomotor (CN III), abducens (CN VI) and nasociliary (CN V) nerves whilst the trochlear (CN IV), lacrimal, frontal and infraorbital (all CN V) remain outside the cone. The orbit and its contents receive a complex innervation of motor, sensory and autonomic nerves, which are listed below in Figure 2.74.

Applied anatomy

The cone of extra-ocular muscles forms an incomplete boundary, which helps to distinguish between retrobulbar and peribulbar

Figure 2.74
Innervation of the orbit and its contents

Modality	Nerve	Innervation
Motor	Oculomotor (CN III)	Superior rectus
		Medial rectus
		Inferior oblique
	Trochlear (CN IV)	Superior oblique
	Abducens (CN VI)	Lateral rectus
	Facial (CN VII)	Orbicularis oculi
Sensory	Trigeminal (CN V)	
	Ophthalmic division	
	Supratrochlear	Skin/conjunctiva upper lid
	Supraorbital	Skin/conjunctiva upper lid
	Long ciliary	Cornea, iris, ciliary muscle
	Nasociliary/infratrochlear	Inner eyelids, inner canthus
	Lacrimal	Lateral canthus, gland, outer lid, conjunctiva
	Maxillary division	
	Infraorbital	Lower lid, nasolacrimal duct
	Zygomatic	Lateral wall of orbit
Autonomic	Sympathetic long and short ciliary nerves from superior cervical ganglion	Iris dilation
	Para-sympathetic fibres from CN III	Iris constriction

Figure 2.75
Sagittal section of orbit showing Tenon's capsule

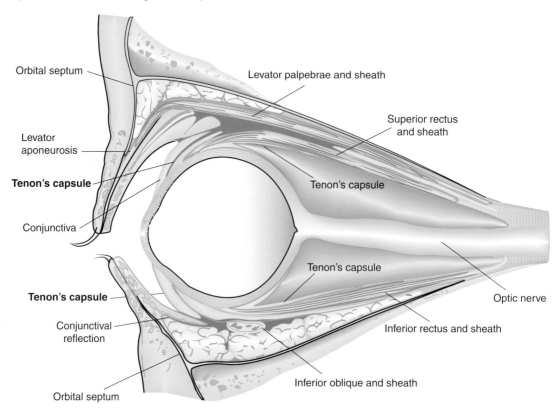

Orbital septum

Levator palpebrae and sheath

Superior rectus and sheath

Levator aponeurosis

Tenon's capsule

Tenon's capsule

Conjunctiva

Tenon's capsule

Tenon's capsule

Optic nerve

Conjunctival reflection

Inferior rectus and sheath

Orbital septum

Inferior oblique and sheath

blocks. With the former the local anaesthetic solution is injected within the cone whilst with the latter, it is injected outside the cone. In practice, there is no complete anatomical boundary between the intra- and extra-conal space, and local anaesthetic diffuses freely between the two.

With any sharp needle technique there is a risk of damage to the globe and therefore it is necessary to know its axial length. The average length is 24 mm but in myopic patients it may be greater than this (up to 33 mm) and the sclera may be correspondingly thinner. Peribulbar and retrobulbar blocks are therefore not recommended if the axial length is greater than 25 mm.

The technique of single quadrant sub-Tenon's block was first described in 1993, and has rapidly become popular for ophthalmic surgery. Tenon's capsule is a thin membrane, which surrounds the globe and attaches anteriorly to the conjunctiva a few millimetres from the limbus (Figure 2.75). Local anaesthetic is introduced between the sclera and Tenon's

capsule, using a *blunt* cannula, to block the sensory nerve supply to the globe. Larger volumes (up to 5 ml) track along the extra-ocular muscles and also escape into the anterior retrobulbar space, to produce a degree of motor block.

Indications

Corneal/conjunctival surgery

Minor surgery to the cornea, sclera and conjunctiva can be carried out under topical anaesthesia alone or in combination with a subconjunctival injection. This might include intra-ocular pressure measurement, removal of foreign bodies, excision of pterygium, irrigation of the lacrimal duct and removal of sutures. Surgical and laser correction of myopia (radial keratotomy) may be undertaken using topical anaesthesia. It is possible to perform cataract surgery under topical anaesthesia alone in some selected patients, with the increasing use of phaco-emulsification through a small limbic incision and the development of foldable intra-ocular lenses.

Intra-ocular surgery

Extracapsular and phaco-emulsification cataract surgery and glaucoma surgery require sensory blockade of the globe and conjunctiva, with some motor blockade of the extra-ocular and orbicularis oculi muscles. Peribulbar, retrobulbar or sub-Tenon's techniques are all suitable for these procedures, producing a dilated pupil, a low intra-ocular pressure and an immobile (akinetic) globe.

Extra-ocular surgery

Squint surgery can be performed with a regional technique but since the patients are predominantly children, general anaesthesia is usually more appropriate. However peribulbar, sub-Tenon's or topical anaesthesia can be used for post-operative analgesia.

Regional anaesthesia for ophthalmology

Topical anaesthesia

Surface landmarks Cornea, conjunctival reflection.
Patient position Supine with the head supported on single pillow/cushion.
Technique Instruct the patient to look straight ahead and hold the eyelids open with the forefinger and middle finger of one hand (Figure 2.76). Drop one or two drops of local anaesthetic solution onto the cornea, which will become anaesthetised almost instantly.
Tetracaine and lidocaine cause marked stinging; therefore benoxinate or proxymetacaine, which are virtually painless, should be instilled first.

Figure 2.76
Topical anaesthesia

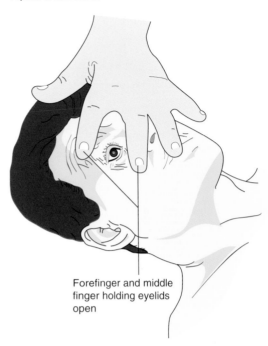

Forefinger and middle finger holding eyelids open

Blocks for intra-ocular surgery

Retrobulbar or peribulbar?

Knapp first described the retrobulbar approach in 1884 and it became the mainstay of ophthalmic regional anaesthesia until recently superseded by more modern techniques. Historically, retrobulbar injections were performed with long (31–50 mm) needles, and a small volume (2 ml) of local anaesthetic solution deposited within the muscle cone at the apex of the orbit. This technique is associated with a significant incidence of serious ocular and systemic side effects, and also requires a separate facial nerve block. For these reasons this technique is not recommended, and will not be described further.

The peribulbar technique was described in 1986, in an attempt to reduce the risk of serious complications of retrobulbar injections. It has become increasingly popular as an alternative and safer block with less risk of serious complications.

Modified retrobulbar injections can be performed with a 25 mm needle, where the local anaesthetic solution is deposited in the anterior intra-conal space and will eventually diffuse out

Agent	Concn (%)	Volume	Onset	Dur (min)
benoxinate	0.4	drops	rapid	5
proxymetacaine	0.5	drops	rapid	5
tetracaine	1	drops	rapid	15
lidocaine	2	drops	rapid	15

Figure 2.77
Retrobulbar block, cross-sectional view (distribution of solution)

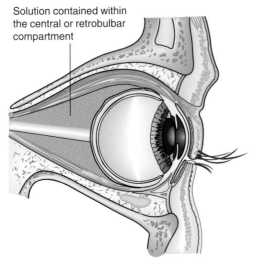

Solution contained within the central or retrobulbar compartment

Figure 2.78
Peribulbar block, cross-sectional view (distribution of solution)

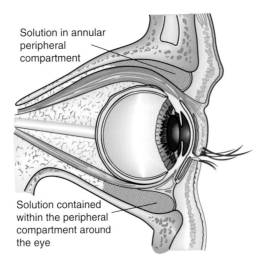

Solution in annular peripheral compartment

Solution contained within the peripheral compartment around the eye

Figure 2.79
Complications of ophthalmic regional anaesthesia

Complication	Cause
Retrobulbar haemorrhage	Intra-conal vessel trauma
Unconsciousness and cadiorespiratory collapse	Intradural cuff injection Vasovagal syncope Local anaesthetic toxicity
Blindness/optic atrophy	Retinal vein/artery injection
	Retrobulbar haemorrhage
Retinal detachment	Globe penetration
Ocular muscle paresis	Intramuscular injection Drug toxicity

branches of the facial nerve to orbicularis oculi muscle, rendering a separate facial nerve block unnecessary. Ocular and systemic complications can occur with either technique (Figure 2.79) and intravenous cannulation is recommended prior to any sharp needle technique.

Subconjunctival block

Subconjunctival injection of very dilute local anaesthetic solutions is painless, and significantly decreases the pain of further injections. This technique can therefore be used either to supplement topical anaesthesia or as a preliminary injection prior to a peribulbar or retrobulbar injection.
Surface landmarks Lateral corneoscleral junction (lateral limbus), lateral canthus, inferior conjunctival reflection.
Patient position Reclining or supine with their gaze fixed straight ahead.
Technique Anaesthetise the cornea and conjunctiva with topical drops as described above and then introduce a 27G or 30G needle through the conjunctival reflection halfway between the lateral limbus and the lateral canthus, towards the floor of the orbit and tangential to the globe. Inject 1–2 ml of local anaesthetic, at a depth of 10–15 mm, after careful aspiration (Figure 2.80).

of the cone into the extra-conal space (Figure 2.77). A peribulbar injection is also performed with a 25 mm needle; the local anaesthetic is deposited outside the cone and slowly diffuses into the intra-conal space (Figure 2.78). The peribulbar technique requires a larger volume of local anaesthetic and has a longer onset time than a retrobulbar injection but it causes smaller rises in intra-ocular pressure. With both techniques, local anaesthetic diffuses anteriorly through the orbital septum, and effectively blocks the terminal

Agent	Concn (%)	Volume (ml)	Onset (min)	Dur (min)
Lidocaine in balanced salt solution	0.2	1–2	2	30

Figure 2.80
Subconjunctival injection

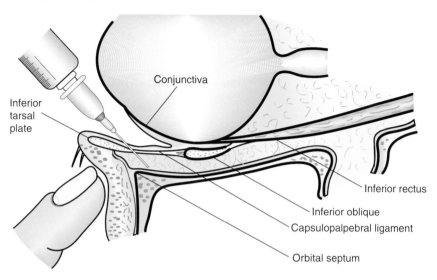

Inferior
tarsal
plate

Conjunctiva

Inferior rectus

Inferior oblique

Capsulopalpebral ligament

Orbital septum

Peribulbar block

Surface landmarks Lateral corneoscleral junction (lateral limbus), lateral canthus, inferior conjunctival reflection, medial canthus, caruncle.
Patient position Reclining or supine with their gaze fixed straight ahead.
Technique Anaesthetise the cornea and conjunctiva as described above and then introduce a 25G, 25 mm (1 inch) needle through the conjunctival reflection halfway between the lateral limbus and the lateral canthus, towards the floor of the orbit and tangential to the globe (Figure 2.81). When the needle touches bone, re-direct so that the needle is parallel to the floor of the orbit, beyond the equator of the globe at a depth of 25 mm. After careful aspiration, slowly inject 5 ml of chosen mixture and closely observe the globe and surrounding structures. Only a minority of patients will have a complete motor and sensory block after a single injection, and a supplementary block can be administered to complete the technique.

The superonasal quadrant should not be used for supplementary injections as it contains a large number of blood vessels and carries a high risk of intravascular injection or haemorrhage.

The second injection is usually made with the same needle, through the conjunctiva at the medial canthus, medial to the caruncle and

Figure 2.81
Needle insertion points, for peri- and retrobulbar blocks

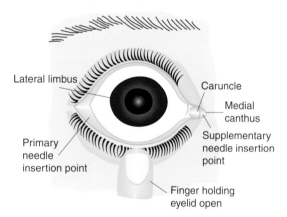

Lateral limbus

Caruncle

Medial canthus

Supplementary needle insertion point

Primary needle insertion point

Finger holding eyelid open

parallel to the medial wall of the orbit. At a depth of 25 mm, inject up to 5 ml of local anaesthetic solution after careful aspiration (Figure 2.81). Injections at this site are always peribulbar or outside the muscle cone. Finally apply a pad and a Honan's balloon inflated to 30 mmHg for 5 min, to disperse the local anaesthetic and reduce intra-ocular pressure (Figures 2.82 and 2.83).

As a consequence of the large volumes used, the local anaesthetic solution diffuses anteriorly through the orbital septum and penetrates the eyelids directly; therefore there

Figure 2.82
Peribulbar block, cross-sectional view

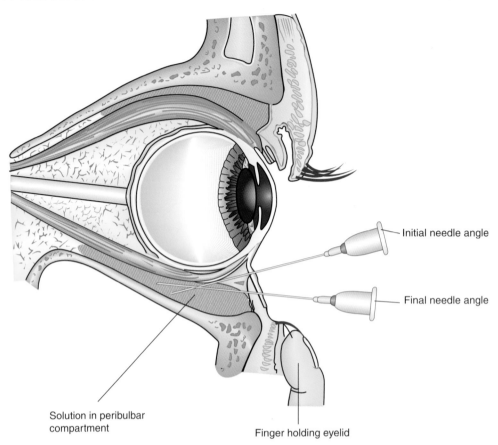

Initial needle angle

Final needle angle

Solution in peribulbar compartment

Finger holding eyelid

Figure 2.83
Medial peribulbar injection, right eye viewed from above

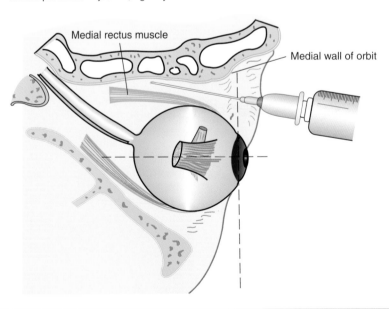

Medial rectus muscle

Medial wall of orbit

is no need for a separate injection into the facial nerve branches.

The most commonly used solution is 2% lidocaine with or without adrenaline, however bupivacaine can be added to prolong the anaesthetic and analgesic effect. Hyaluronidase 5–30 units/ml is usually added to the mixture to aid spread through the periorbital tissues.

Retrobulbar block

An anterior retrobulbar block may be performed in a similar way to the peribulbar block described above, using a 25G, 25 mm needle. The landmarks for the first injection are identical (Figure 2.81) but the needle should be re-directed more cranially once past the equator of the globe, so that the final position of the needle is intra-conal (Figure 2.84). Less volume

Agent	Concn (%)	Volume (ml)	Onset (min)	Dur
lidocaine	2	10	5	45 min
lidocaine + adrenaline	2 (1:200,000)	10	5	1.5 h
bupivacaine	0.5	5	10	4 h
bupivacaine + lidocaine	2	5		
bupivacaine	0.75	2	10	4 h
bupivacaine + lidocaine	2	8		

Figure 2.84
Retrobulbar block, cross-sectional view

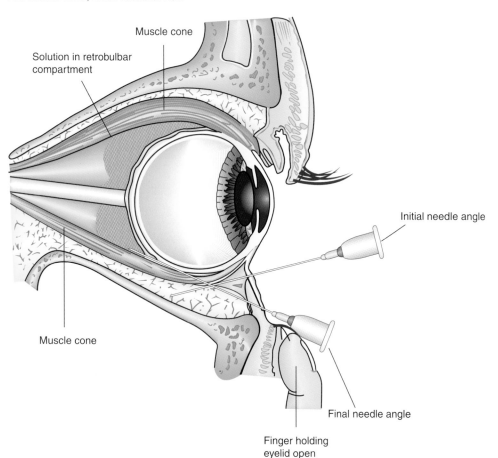

Muscle cone

Solution in retrobulbar compartment

Initial needle angle

Muscle cone

Final needle angle

Finger holding eyelid open

Figure 2.85
Sterile equipment required for sub-Tenon's block

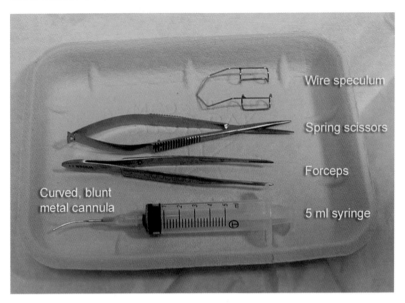

Figure 2.86
Sub-Tenon's technique (right eye)

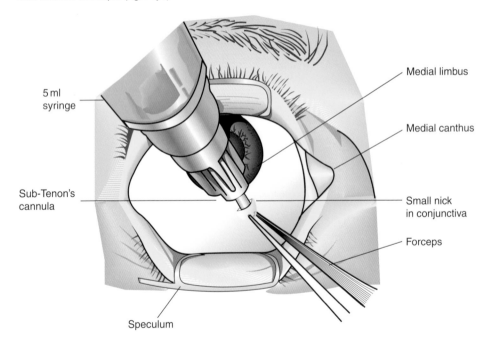

(3 ml) is required in this position, to prevent large increases in intra-ocular pressure. A second medial injection is usually required to block the orbicularis oculi muscles. The solutions used are similar but the total volumes are less (5–7 ml).

Sub-Tenon's block

Surface landmarks Inferomedial corneoscleral junction (inferomedial limbus), inferomedial conjunctival reflection.

Patient position Reclining or supine. To block the right eye stand above the patients head and for the left eye stand at their left side.

Technique Anaesthetise the cornea and conjunctiva as previously described, and also instil 2 drops of 1 in 10,000 adrenaline to aid conjunctival haemostasis. As this is a surgical technique, aqueous betadine solution is instilled into the eye and used to clean the eyelids. The operator should wear sterile gloves. The list of surgical instruments required is listed in Figure 2.85.

Insert the speculum underneath the eyelids, and ask the patient to look upwards and outwards. In the inferomedial quadrant, midway between the limbus and the conjunctival reflection, grasp the conjunctiva with the forceps. Make a small nick in the conjunctiva with the scissors, and with gentle blunt dissection identify the underlying sclera, which should appear white with tiny overlying blood vessels. Attach the 5 ml syringe of local anaesthetic to the cannula. Introduce the blunt metal cannula into the conjunctival incision with its curve following the curve of the globe. Gently advance the cannula using hydro-dissection to overcome any resistance, until the cannula is inserted almost to its full length and then inject up to 5 ml of solution (Figure 2.86).

If there is immediate ballooning of the conjunctiva and escape of fluid from the incision then the cannula is too superficial. Ensure that both Tenon's capsule and the conjunctiva have been incised, using further dissection. Once the injection is completed, remove the speculum, close the eyelids and apply gentle digital pressure or a Honan's balloon for up to 5 min.

This technique provides excellent anaesthesia and akinesia without the ocular and systemic risks of a sharp needle technique. It is particularly indicated for myopic patients, or those with a blind fellow eye. A degree of conjunctival oedema (chemosis) and subconjunctival haemorrhage is common, but does not interfere with surgery or cause the patient any discomfort post-operatively.

Hyaluronidase 5–30 units/ml should be added to the above solutions.

Agent	Concn (%)	Vol (ml)	Onset (min)	Dur
lidocaine	2	5	2	45 min
lidocaine + adrenaline	2 (1:200,000)	5	2	1.5 h

The head, neck and airway

Introduction

The head and neck have a complex innervation from both cranial and peripheral nerves and there is considerable overlap of adjacent nerve territories. This makes it difficult to decide which specific nerve blocks are required and whether they are practical and appropriate. The superficial sensory nerves are easy to locate and block and are used in plastic and cosmetic surgery. Major surgery to the head and neck under regional anaesthesia is not practical except for surgery on the carotid artery. Some chronic pain states may respond to diagnostic and neurolytic cranial and peripheral nerve blocks.

Discrete nerve blocks of the pharynx and larynx (CN V, IX and X) have traditionally been used for bronchoscopy and awake intubation of the trachea but have been largely superseded by topical anaesthesia supplemented by cricothyroid membrane puncture and intra-tracheal spray.

Anatomy

Cranial nerves

Some cranial nerves have specialised somatic and autonomic functions and are not amenable to practical nerve blockade. CN III, IV and VI are routinely blocked during ophthalmic regional techniques but otherwise, the trigeminal nerve (CN V), which innervates the skin of the anterior two-thirds of the scalp and face (Figure 2.87) is the only cranial nerve with terminal sensory branches that are easy and practical to block.

Trigeminal nerve

The trigeminal nerve has three divisions – ophthalmic (V1), maxillary (V2) and mandibular (V3), which terminate in a number of cutaneous nerves. Of these, the supraorbital and supra-trochlear (V1), the infraorbital, zygomaticofacial and zygomaticotemporal (V2) and the mental (V3) can be blocked by discrete injection as they emerge from bony foraminae.

The *supraorbital* and *supratrochlear* nerves emerge close together on the superior and

Figure 2.87
Nerve territories of the terminal nerves

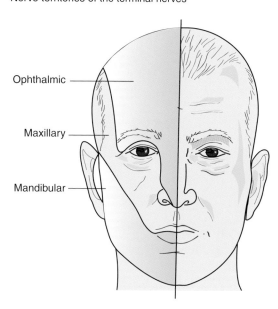

Ophthalmic

Maxillary

Mandibular

superiomedial borders of the orbit respectively, to supply the skin of the upper eyelid and lower forehead (supratrochlear) and the forehead and the anterior aspect of the scalp as far back as the vertex (supraorbital). The *infraorbital* nerve emerges from its foramen about 1 cm below the midpoint of the lower orbital border. It innervates the skin of the lower eyelid, side of the nose, cheek and upper lip. The *mental* nerve emerges from the mental foramen in the mandible to innervate the skin of the chin and lower lip (Figure 2.87).

The *zygomaticofacial* and *zygomaticotemporal* nerves emerge from small foraminae in the zygoma, near the lateral orbital margin, to supply the skin of the cheek, temple and adjoining scalp. The *auriculotemporal* nerve emerges from behind the temporomandibular joint and accompanies the superficial temporal artery. It innervates the skin of the temple, the tragus and part of the helix of the ear.

Applied anatomy

The supraorbital, infraorbital and mental foraminae lie in the same vertical plane, which runs through the pupil when the eye is in the mid-position. They innervate the anterior

Figure 2.88
Cranial and peripheral nerves innervating the side of the head and neck

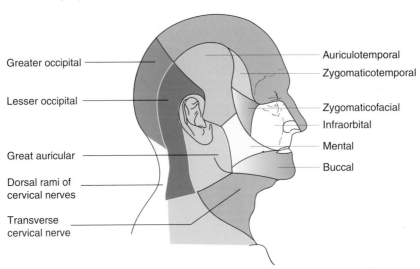

aspect of the face and are usually blocked in combination for minor reconstructive/plastic surgery of the face.

The zygomaticofacial and zygomatico-temporal nerves together with the auriculotemporal innervate the side of the face and form a boundary with the peripheral nerves of the head and neck that innervate the rest of the ear, scalp and neck.

Cervical nerves

The *dorsal rami* of cervical nerves 1–4 innervate the posterior aspect of the scalp as far forward as the vertex, the inferior and posterior surfaces of the ear and the neck. The dorsal rami of C1 and 2 are larger than the ventral rami and form the suboccipital (C1, motor only) and greater occipital (C2) nerves which supplies the scalp. The dorsal rami of C3 and 4 innervate the skin of the back of the neck (Figure 2.88).

Greater occipital nerve

The greater occipital nerve pierces the trapezius muscle about 2 cm lateral to the occipital protuberance to become subcutaneous. The occipital artery accompanies it and is a convenient landmark. It innervates the scalp as far anterior as the vertex and often communicates with the lesser occipital nerve.

The *ventral rami* of C1–4 combine to form the cervical plexus anterior to the scalenus medius

muscle and deep to the sternomastoid muscle and internal jugular vein. The plexus gives rise to superficial (sensory) and deep (motor) branches, although the phrenic nerve (C3–5), a branch of the deep plexus, also has efferent visceral sensory nerve fibres.

Superficial cervical plexus

The superficial branches of the plexus (C2–4) emerge from behind the posterior border of sternomastoid muscle at its midpoint (Figure 2.89). They penetrate the deep cervical fascia and radiate out subcutaneously to supply the ear and surrounding skin of the scalp and face (lesser occipital and greater auricular nerves), the skin of the neck and the shoulder and the uppermost parts of the chest wall (the anterior cutaneous nerve and the supraclavicular nerves).

Deep cervical plexus

The cervical roots 1–4 emerge from the intervertebral foraminae, lying in the grooves (sulci) of the transverse processes before combining to form the plexus. At this level the roots are between the middle and anterior scalene muscles (similar to the brachial plexus) and an approach to the roots is, in effect, a cervical paravertebral block. The deep, motor branches curl round scalenus anterior and pass medially, deep to sternomastoid while the superficial branches continue laterally to

Figure 2.89
Superficial cervical plexus

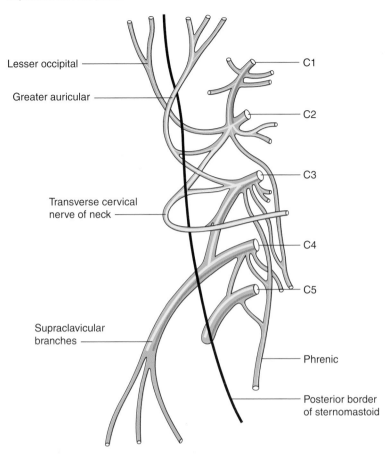

Lesser occipital

Greater auricular

Transverse cervical
nerve of neck

Supraclavicular
branches

C1

C2

C3

C4

C5

Phrenic

Posterior border
of sternomastoid

emerge at the midpoint of the posterior border
of sternomastoid.

Applied anatomy

There are few indications for a deep approach to
the cervical plexus as any injection made at the
level of the roots will produce phrenic nerve
paralysis and may spread to the more distal
cervical nerves causing a partial brachial plexus
block. Limiting cervical plexus blocks to the
superficial branches achieves complete sensory
blockade without motor deficit and the
superficial plexus can be blocked by a single
injection whereas the deep plexus requires
separate injections at the level of each transverse
process. Other potential complications of the
deep approach to the cervical plexus include
vertebral artery injection causing rapid systemic
toxicity, injection through the dural cuff of a

cervical nerve root to produce high spinal block
and recurrent laryngeal nerve block.

Indications

Surgery to the head and neck can be carried out
under local anaesthesia alone or under light
general anaesthesia supplemented by local
anaesthetic techniques for post-operative
analgesia.

Surgery of the scalp

Wounds of the scalp can be repaired under a
combination of nerve blocks according to the
position of the wound. Posterior to the ears, the
greater and lesser occipital and great auricular
nerves need to be blocked. Anterior to the ears,
the supratrochlear, supraorbital and
auriculotemporal nerves need to be blocked.

Surgery of the face

Superficial surgery to the face can be accomplished with discrete nerve blocks of the appropriate nerve(s), supplemented with local infiltration.

Surgery of the ear

Operations on the pinna can be carried out with auriculotemporal nerve block anteriorly and greater auricular and lesser occipital nerve blocks posteriorly.

Surgery of the neck

Superficial surgery only requires superficial cervical plexus blockade. Bilateral blocks are needed for midline operations such as tracheostomy and thyroidectomy and may need to be reinforced with local infiltration. Deep cervical plexus block has been advocated for these procedures but in view of the need for bilateral blocks and the risk of bilateral phrenic nerve blockade, this is not recommended.

The main indication for blocking the deep branches of the cervical plexus is carotid artery surgery. Regional anaesthesia is widely used for carotid endarterectomy as it produces a favourable outcome for this operation compared to general anaesthesia.

Techniques

Superficial cervical plexus block (Figure 2.90)

Surface landmarks Posterior border of sternomastoid (PBS), cricoid cartilage (CC).
Patient position Supine with the head turned slightly to the opposite side, as in Figure 2.90.
Technique Draw a line laterally from the cricoid cartilage to cross the posterior border of the sternomastoid muscle at the midpoint between the sternal notch and the mastoid process. The superficial branches of the plexus usually emerge from deep to the sternomastoid muscle at this point (a). If the posterior border is difficult to identify, ask the patient to raise their head from the pillow slightly with it turned away from the side to be blocked. Insert a 22G short bevel needle immediately behind the muscle at right angles to the skin until it 'pops' through the cervical fascia (b). If the needle is in the correct tissue plane, an injection of 10 ml of local anaesthetic will distend the deep tissue plane along the posterior border of the muscle.

Agent	Concn (%)	Volume (ml)	Onset (min)	Dur (h)
l-bupiv	0.5	10	20	12
lido	1	10	10	4

Deep cervical plexus block (Figure 2.91)

Surface landmarks Mastoid process, C6 transverse process (Chassaignac's tubercle).
Patient position Head on low pillow, turned to opposite side from block.
Technique Draw a line between the mastoid process and the transverse process of C6 at the level of the cricoid cartilage. Approximately 1.5 cm caudad to the mastoid process gently palpate the neck just posterior to the line and feel for the transverse process of C2. Mark this point and move a further 1.5 cm caudad and repeat the process for the transverse process of C3. Finally, move a further 1.5 cm caudad along the line and palpate the transverse process of C4, which is usually level with the midpoint of the posterior border of the sternomastoid

Figure 2.90
Superficial cervical plexus block

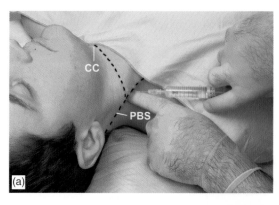
(a)

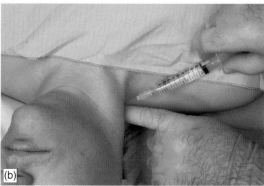
(b)

muscle (a). Raise a wheal at each of the points marked and insert a 3.5 cm 22G needle perpendicularly to the skin at each point (b). Carefully direct the needle towards the transverse process aiming posteriorly (dorsally) and slightly caudad, being especially careful not to direct the needle medially. On contact with the transverse process, immobilise the needle, confirm negative aspiration of blood and cerebrospinal fluid (CSF) and then slowly inject 3–5 ml of local anaesthetic checking with frequent aspiration to avoid intravascular or central nervous injection. Repeat at each level (c).

Agent	Concn (%)	Volume (ml)	Onset (min)	Dur (h)
l-bupiv	0.5	3–5 per level	5	4–6

Figure 2.91
Deep approach to the cervical plexus

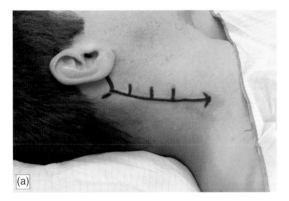

(a)

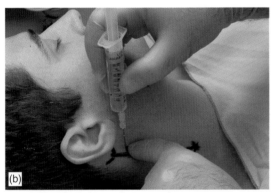

(b)

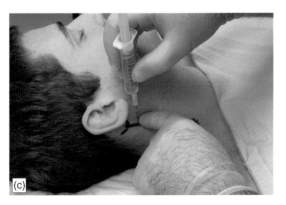

(c)

Greater and lesser occipital nerve block

The lesser occipital nerve and the greater auricular nerve can be blocked with a cervical plexus block or they can be blocked separately.
Surface landmarks Greater occipital protuberance, mastoid process, posterior occipital artery.
Patient position Sitting up.
Technique Palpate the occipital protuberance and the mastoid process and define a line between them. Insert a 25G needle subcutaneously, 2 cm lateral to the occipital protuberance, aiming along the line between the bony landmarks (the pulsation of the artery may be palpable at this point). Inject 4–5 ml of solution at the point of insertion and a further 3–4 ml subcutaneously by advancing the needle towards the mastoid process to block the lesser occipital nerve (Figure 2.92).

Agent	Concn (%)	Volume (ml)	Onset (min)	Dur (h)
l-bupiv	0.25	7–9	10	6
lido	1	7–9	6	4

Figure 2.92
Greater and lesser occipital nerve block

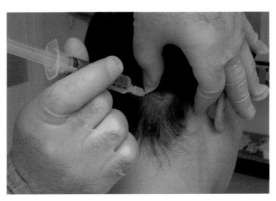

Figure 2.93
Great auricular nerve block

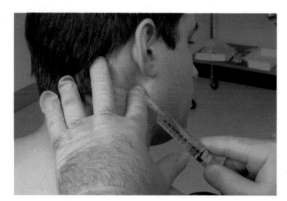

Figure 2.94
Auriculotemporal nerve block

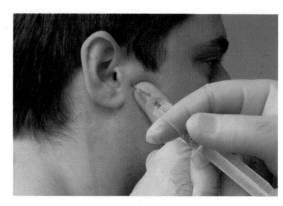

Greater auricular nerve block

Surface landmarks Mastoid process.
Patient position Sitting up.
Technique Turn the head away from the side to be blocked to expose the mastoid process. Infiltrate 7–10 ml of solution along the posterior aspect of the mastoid process using a 25G needle (Figure 2.93).

Agent	Concn (%)	Volume (ml)	Onset (min)	Dur (h)
l-bupiv	0.25	7–10	10	6–8

Figure 2.95
Zygomaticofacial and zygomaticotemporal nerve blocks

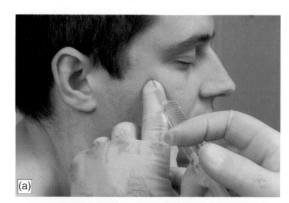

(a)

Auriculotemporal nerve block

Surface landmarks Superficial temporal artery, temporomandibular joint, tragus of ear.
Patient position Head on pillow turned slightly away from side to be blocked.
Technique Palpate the temporal artery just above the temporomandibular joint. Insert a 23G needle at right angles to the skin between the pulsation of the artery and the tragus and after careful negative aspiration, inject 2–3 ml of solution (Figure 2.94).

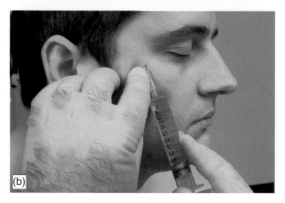

(b)

Agent	Concn (%)	Volume (ml)	Onset (min)	Dur (h)
lido	1	4–6	5–6	3–4
l-bupiv	0.25	4–6	10	4–6

Zygomaticofacial and zygomaticotemporal nerve blocks (Figure 2.95)

These nerves have limited territories and are usually blocked in combination.
Surface landmarks Zygomaticofacial foramen, lateral border of orbit.

Patient position Lying with head turned away from side to be blocked.

Technique Palpate the zygomaticofacial foramen 1 cm or so below the lateral border of the orbit. Use a 25G needle to make a subcutaneous injection of 2–3 ml of solution around the branches of the nerve as they emerge from the foramen (a) and then re-direct the needle subcutaneously along the lateral border of the orbit and inject a further 2–3 ml to block the zygomaticotemporal nerve (b).

Agent	Concn (%)	Volume (ml)	Onset (min)	Dur (h)
lido	1	4–6	5	3–4
l-bupiv	0.25	4–6	10	4–6

Anterior facial nerve blocks

The three foraminae for the mental nerve, infraorbital nerve and supraorbital blocks all lie in the same plane which passes through the pupil when the eye is held in its midpoint resting position (Figure 2.96).

Mental nerve block

Surface landmarks Mental foramen.
Patient position Head on pillow looking straight ahead
Technique Palpate the mental foramen of the mandible and introduce a 25G needle subcutaneously towards the foramen (Figure 2.97). It is not necessary to enter the foramen. An injection of 2–3 ml close to the foramen is sufficient.

Agent	Concn (%)	Volume (ml)	Onset (min)	Dur (h)
l-bupiv	0.25	3	10	6
lido	1	3	6	4

Infraorbital nerve block

Surface landmarks Infraorbital foramen.
Patient position As for mental block.
Technique Palpate the infraorbital foramen, approximately 1 cm below the midpoint of the lower border of the orbit and 1 cm lateral to the nose. Insert a 25G needle subcutaneously towards the foramen and inject 2–3 ml of

Figure 2.96
Anterior facial foraminae

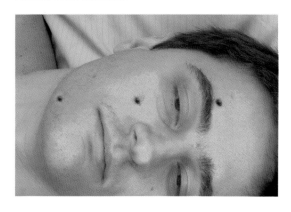

Figure 2.97
Mental nerve block, anterior view

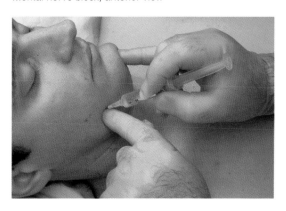

Figure 2.98
Infraorbital nerve block

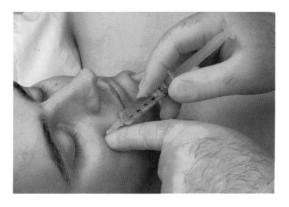

solution around the outlet of the foramen (Figure 2.98). Do not introduce the needle into the nerve canal as the nerve and the floor of the orbit can be damaged.

Agent	Concn (%)	Volume (ml)	Onset (min)	Dur (h)
l-bupiv	0.25	3	10	6
lido	1	3	6	4

Supraorbital and supratrochlear nerve blocks (Figure 2.99)

These nerves are usually blocked together because of their proximity and overlapping territories.

Surface landmarks Supraorbital notch, bridge of nose.

Patient position As for mental block.

Technique Palpate the supraorbital notch, at the midpoint of the superior border of the orbit and insert a 25G needle subcutaneously so that the tip just touches the periosteum of the frontal bone. Withdraw the needle very slightly and slowly inject 3–4 ml of solution (a). Re-angle medially and inject a further 2–3 ml of solution as a subcutaneous 'sausage' while advancing the needle medially along the orbital border as far as the bridge of the nose (b).

Figure 2.99
(a) Supraorbital and (b) Supratrochlear nerve block

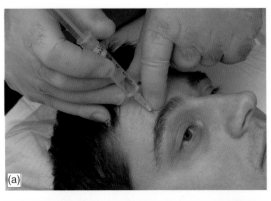

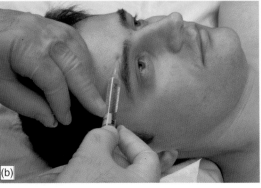

For bilateral anaesthesia, use a midpoint injection on the bridge of the nose, through a skin wheal of local anaesthetic. Direct the needle subcutaneously towards the supraorbital notch on one side and inject 5–7 ml of solution continuously as the needle is advanced 1 cm beyond the notch. Withdraw the needle and re-direct towards the other supraorbital notch and repeat the injection.

Agent	Concn (%)	Volume (ml)	Onset (min)	Dur (h)
lido	1	5–7	10	3–4
l-bupiv	0.25	5–7	15	6–8

Local anaesthesia of the upper airway

The mucosal surfaces of the nose, mouth, naso and oropharynx, glottis, larynx and trachea can be anaesthetised by a combination of topical anaesthesia and discrete nerve blocks. Traditionally there was more emphasis on specific nerve blocks either by needle injection techniques or by transmucosal absorption of local anaesthetic from pledgets placed within the airway. Recently, with advances in fibreoptic bronchoscopy and awake oral or nasal intubation there has been a move towards the use of topically applied local anaesthetic solution, although nerve blocks are still used to supplement topical anaesthesia when indicated.

Anatomy

The airway is innervated with a complex nerve supply from three different cranial nerves. The *trigeminal nerve* supplies the nose, nasopharynx, palate (V2) and anterior aspect of tongue (V3). The *glossopharyngeal nerve* supplies the oropharynx, posterior aspect of tongue and soft palate. The *superior laryngeal* and *recurrent laryngeal nerves* are branches of the vagus nerve and supply motor, secretomotor and sensory fibres to the airway below the epiglottis (Figure 2.100). They both arise from the inferior ganglion of the vagus nerve, just above the hyoid bone. The superior laryngeal nerve emerges beneath the inferior edge of the greater cornu of the hyoid before it divides into the internal and external branches. The recurrent laryngeal nerve loops under the arch of the aorta before ascending to innervate the larynx.

Applied anatomy

All the nerves innervating the airway contribute secretomotor, sensory and motor control over the protective relexes of the airway – the gag, cough and glottic closure reflexes. Therefore any local anaesthetic technique will block these important reflexes and the patient's airway will be at risk of aspiration until the reflexes recover fully.

Indications

- Fibreoptic endoscopy of the upper respiratory tract and major airways

Figure 2.100
Nerve supply to the upper airway

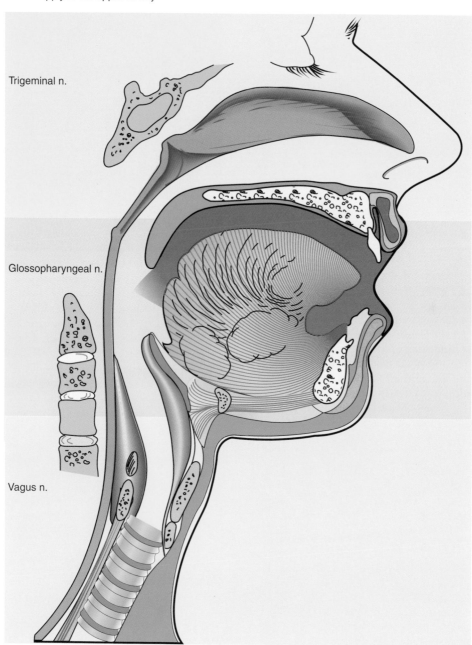

Trigeminal n.

Glossopharyngeal n.

Vagus n.

- Awake intubation of trachea in patients with difficult airways due to variant anatomy, trauma or disease
- Intubation may be via the nose and nasopharynx or via the mouth and oropharynx

Technique

Local anaesthesia of the upper airway is largely comprised of topical anaesthesia, supplemented where appropriate by superior laryngeal nerve block and transtracheal anaesthesia.

Awake intubation of the airway requires particular emphasis on explanation and patient preparation and usually some sedation to ensure that the patient is calm and co-operative. An antisialogogic injection is commonly recommended (glycopyrrolate 200 mcg i.v.) in addition to sedation.

Topical

Spraying

Surface landmarks The mouth and oropharynx.
Patient position Sitting up with the mouth open maximally.
Technique Spray 4 metered puffs of lidocaine (10 mg per spray) from a commercially available 10% solution aerosol spray onto the tongue and wait a few minutes for it to take effect (Figure 2.101). Depress the tongue and spray a further four puffs onto the posterior part of the tongue and pharynx. Other methods of producing the same effect include disposable 4% solution sprays, nebulisers, atomisers and getting the patient to gargle a solution of local anaesthetic. Whichever method is used it is important to ensure that the maximum dose of lidocaine is not exceeded and that any surplus anaesthetic is spat out and not swallowed by the patient.

Direct application

Surface landmarks External nares of the nose.
Patient position Sitting up with the head tilted back.
Technique Soak two cotton tipped swabs in 2% lidocaine and gently introduce one into chosen nostril and then the other beyond the first one into the nasopharynx. Leave for 5 min.

Figure 2.101
Topical anaesthesia of the airway

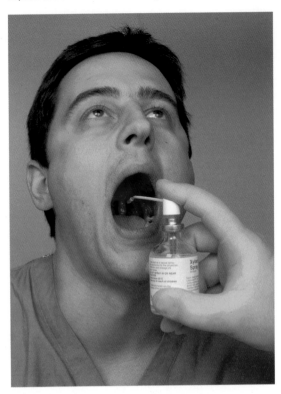

Agent	Concn (%)	Volume (ml)	Onset (min)	Dur (h)
lido	2–4	Variable	5	30–60

Other direct application techniques include placing soaked cotton tipped swabs into the tonsillar fauces to anaesthetise the glossopharyngeal nerve and the superior laryngeal nerve is similarly anaesthetised by placing pledgets soaked in 2% lidocaine into each pyriform fossa with Krause forceps.

Once the nasal or oral mucosa is anaesthetised, lidocaine can be directly applied to the rest of the airway through the working channel of the fibreoptic bronchoscope or discrete nerve block techniques may be used.

Nerve blockade
Superior laryngeal nerve block

Surface landmarks Hyoid bone, thyroid cartilage.

Figure 2.102
Superior laryngeal nerve block

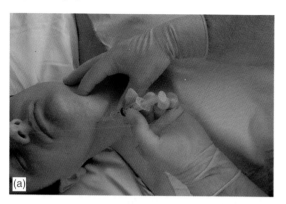

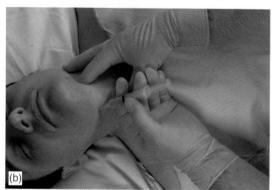

Figure 2.103
Transtracheal block

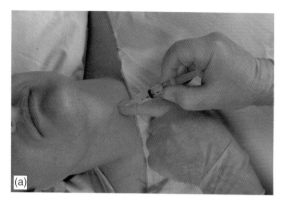

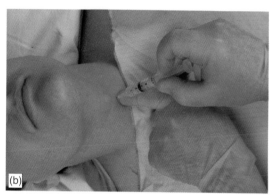

Patient position Supine with the head extended.
Technique Palpate the hyoid cartilage just cephalad to the thyroid cartilage. Displace the hyoid slightly towards the side to be blocked and insert a 25G, 2.5 cm needle just under the inferior border of the hyoid and inject 2–3 ml of 1% lidocaine, moving the needle gently in and out through the thyrohyoid membrane (Figure 2.102). Repeat on the other side.

Agent	Concn (%)	Volume (ml)	Onset (min)	Dur (h)
lido	1–2	2–3	5	1–3

Transtracheal injection (Figure 2.103)

Surface landmarks Inferior border of thyroid cartilage, cricoid cartilage, cricothyroid membrane.

Patient position As for superior laryngeal nerve block.
Technique Palpate the inferior border of the thyroid cartilage and anaesthetise the overlying skin. Insert a 21G, 2.5 cm needle through the cricothyroid membrane into the lumen of the trachea (a). Ensure that air aspirates freely and then rapidly inject 3–4 ml of 2% lidocaine. This will precipitate brisk coughing which spreads the local anaesthetic throughout the trachea and up into the larynx and vocal cords (b).
Total doses of lidocaine used for topical, direct application and nerve blocks for airway anaesthesia in an average 70 kg adult should not exceed 200 mg.

Agent	Concn (%)	Volume (ml)	Onset (min)	Dur (h)
lido	2–4	3–5	Rapid	60

Continuous peripheral nerve catheter techniques

Introduction

Peripheral nerve block infusions were first described nearly 60 years ago, when Ansbro (1946) used a malleable metal intravenous needle to cannulate the brachial plexus. Catheter techniques are increasingly being used to provide infusions over several days or even weeks for treating a variety of acute and chronic pain conditions and they can be used with most major peripheral nerves. Standard approaches for single-shot techniques are used, although some minor modifications are usually necessary to actually insert the catheter.

Benefits of catheter infusion techniques

Prolonged analgesia

Following major orthopaedic, reconstructive or trauma surgery, severe pain and reflex muscle spasm can significantly delay rehabilitation and the return of full function. Some chronic pain states also cause significant limb dysfunction and the use of catheter infusion techniques can improve outcome from major surgery and chronic pain by providing continuous, prolonged neural blockade.

Patients undergoing major orthopaedic procedures, such as total knee replacement or ligament reconstruction, experience severe pain, despite conventional post-operative analgesia for up to 72 h. These patients may require continuous passive movement and physio-therapy for the first 24–48 h and this treatment is better tolerated if prolonged femoral nerve (and sciatic, if indicated) blockade is used.

Brachial plexus catheter techniques may be used to provide prolonged analgesia after complex reconstruction of the shoulder, elbow, forearm and hand. For post-operative manage-ment of major, unilateral, thoraco-abdominal surgery, interpleural, thoracic and lumbar para-vertebral catheter techniques are used. Breast reconstruction, thoracotomy and renal surgery are all suitable for these techniques. Chronic pain conditions, either due to malignancy, ischaemia or reflex sympathetic dystrophy can be more effectively managed once prolonged analgesia with peripheral nerve catheters has been achieved.

Sympathetic blockade

Many peripheral nerve blocks induce a widespread sympathetic block in the distribution of the nerve(s) affected for the duration of the sensory and motor block. This temporary sympathectomy will improve regional blood flow in the affected area, which may be important in improving areas of critical perfusion for the reconstruction of traumatised limbs or the creation of skin flaps or arterio-venous fistulae. After major vascular surgery, the incidence of graft failure is significantly reduced by regional anaesthesia, due to both improved blood flow to the graft and reduced reflex thrombogenic response following surgery. In patients with ischaemic rest pain of the lower limb, it is often possible to improve the blood supply so that in addition to alleviating the pain, any surgery that may be required can be planned more effectively.

Improved patient management

Effective peripheral nerve blockade will reduce or avoid the need for opioid drugs which can be of great help in managing high-risk patients with significant co-morbidity. Chronic pain may be opioid resistant with the result that high doses of opioids are administered, providing sub-optimal analgesia whilst causing many of the well-recognised side effects. In common with other pain management techniques, multi-modal analgesia using a combination of non-steroidal anti-inflammatory drugs (NSAIDs), paracetamol and small doses of opioids to enhance the effects of the catheter infusion will produce optimal levels of pain control with minimal side effects and risk.

Indications

- acute pain
  - trauma
  - post-operative pain
- chronic pain
  - complex regional pain syndrome (reflex sympathetic dystrophy)
  - phantom pain
- prolonged sympathetic blockade
  - vascular compromise
- terminal cancer pain

Equipment

There have been a number of new developments in needle/catheter design in recent years, as these techniques become more popular. Although it is possible to use equipment that is not specifically designed for perineural catheter placement (intravenous cannulae or catheters), it is preferable to use purpose-designed equipment with short bevel needles and soft-tip catheters, to reduce the risk of nerve injury. There are four basic types of needle/catheter combination:

1. *Catheter over needle*: This combination limits the length of catheter to that of the needle and is only suitable for axillary plexus block or superficial peripheral nerve blockade, at the elbow for instance.
2. *Cannula over needle, catheter through cannula*: There are a wide variety of these kits available with different lengths and calibre of cannula. They are most effective and easy to insert when the needle insertion is parallel, or nearly so, to the axis of the nerve or plexus. When the needle is inserted at 90° to the axis of the nerve, the cannula can be difficult to insert very far without kinking or obstructing.
3. *Catheter through needle*: Where the needle is inserted at an angle to the long axis of the nerve or plexus, needles with a side-opening hole such as a Tuohy or Sprotte are used to encourage the catheter to run alongside the nerve, although success is not always guaranteed. Insulated epidural Tuohy needles have recently become available and are an interesting new development.
4. *Seldinger technique*: Catheter kits based on the Seldinger wire technique are preferable to catheter through needle kits as the needle used to place the wire has a smaller gauge and is less likely to cause local anaesthetic leakage when the catheter is positioned, as the catheter will fit more tightly through the smaller diameter hole, made by the needle, as it is introduced over the wire.

Catheters range in size from 20G to 24G, depending on the site of insertion and should be long enough to allow for them to be tunnelled away from the site of insertion. This may reduce the risk of infection and accidental catheter dislodgement and can make it easier for the patient and their carers to care for the catheter. *Peripheral nerve stimulators* are an essential piece of equipment for accurately locating the nerve trunks or plexus. At present they are used in combination with an insulated needle to allow precise placement of the needle but the insertion of the catheter is still placed 'blind' with no confirmation of its final position unless radiological contrast medium is injected. Perineural catheters that incorporate a stimulating electrode along the length of the catheter assist accurate placement by stimulating the nerve with the tip of the catheter as it is advanced through the needle. However, the catheters are very expensive and as yet there is insufficient experience to justify using them routinely.

Radiological confirmation

The introduction and final positioning of catheters can be confirmed by the use of an image intensifier and a suitable water-soluble X-ray contrast medium.

Peripheral nerve block techniques

Suitable techniques for use with catheters are shown in Figure 2.104.

Standard approaches to most nerves are suitable for inserting catheters, although minor modifications may be necessary. In the majority of cases, inserting a catheter is more technically difficult than the single-shot technique. Figure 2.105 lists a number of practical tips to help improve success rates.

Figure 2.104
Continuous catheter techniques

Technique	Approach
Brachial plexus	Interscalene Subclavian perivascular Vertical infraclavicular Axillary
Paravertebral	Thoracic Lumbar
Interpleural	Interpleural
Femoral nerve	Proximal (psoas compartment, lumbar plexus) Distal (Winnie's '3 in 1')
Sciatic	Transgluteal (Labat) Posterior (lithotomy) Popliteal fossa (lateral or posterior)

Upper limb

The primary site of catheter insertion is the brachial plexus and all major approaches to the plexus (interscalene, subclavian perivascular and axillary) can be used. The vertical infraclavicular approach is a recently described technique and is also suitable for catheter insertion. Each approach uses the anatomical and topographical landmarks of the standard single-shot techniques, although minor modifications are often necessary because of the larger calibre of needle/catheter combination. The interscalene approach is most useful for shoulder and humerus surgery, whilst the axillary or infraclavicular routes are preferable for forearm and hand surgery. Catheters can be used more distally at the elbow and the wrist but these sites have only limited use.

The major practical concern having inserted the catheter is to secure it. The interscalene and axillary approaches are difficult areas to secure the catheter firmly because of the mobility of the neck and arm. Tunnel an axillary catheter distally towards the midpoint of the humerus where the skin is less mobile and apply a firm dressing. For interscalene, subclavian perivascular and infraclavicular approaches, tunnel the catheter onto the anterior chest wall where it is easier to secure.

Lower limb

In contrast to the upper limb, there is no single technique suitable for the lower limb. Due to the separate territories of the two major plexuses and their terminal nerves, it is usually necessary to catheterise both the femoral and sciatic nerves, although a popliteal fossa catheter block is usually sufficient for blockade below the knee.

Plexus blocks

These use a modified approach of the technique described in p 54 of Section 2, Chapter 1, to place a catheter within the psoas muscle compartment. A psoas compartment catheter is usually combined with a sciatic nerve block for proximal lower limb surgery, such as hip joint and femoral shaft surgery.

Nerve blocks

Femoral nerve and proximal sciatic nerve catheters have been in use for about 20 years. More recently, techniques for placing a catheter in the popliteal fossa either via the posterior or lateral route have become popular.

For the femoral nerve, the landmarks are the same as for a standard perivascular (Winnie) '3 in 1' block. An insulated 50 mm 18G Tuohy needle and 20G catheter kit is suitable, as the angle of the needle tip allows the catheter to thread up the femoral nerve sheath easily. For the most reliable proximal placement of a catheter, use a Seldinger wire technique as the wire will often thread right up to the lumbar plexus.

The classic transgluteal (Labat) approach to the sciatic nerve is the best approach for

Figure 2.105
Practical tips for inserting peripheral nerve catheters

1. Try to insert the needle as close to the long axis of the nerve or plexus as possible in order to encourage easier insertion of the catheter. For the brachial plexus, the interscalene and axillary approaches are the best in this regard.

2. Having located the nerve or plexus with the needle, inject 3–5 ml of saline or local anaesthetic to distend the sheath and make it easier to insert the catheter. Some people prefer to inject the entire dose of local anaesthetic at this point to guarantee that they produce an effective block in case they cannot insert the catheter.

3. Insert the catheter 3–4 cm at most; it may be necessary to use a little force to 'persuade' the catheter beyond the tip of the needle. Once it begins to move beyond the needle tip the catheter may run more smoothly. If not, inject a further 3–4 ml via the catheter to distend the sheath slightly before advancing again. Do not try to force the catheter if it does not advance; it will either kink or displace the needle or cannula used to insert it. Instead, try to re-angle the needle or re-orientate the needle bevel before trying to advance the catheter again.

4. Once the catheter is in its final position, inject the main dose of local anaesthetic, if appropriate, or a bolus of saline to ensure that the catheter is patent and the injection is of low resistance. Secure the catheter or tunnel it away from the site of insertion as appropriate and ensure that all the junctions of the catheter and filter are tight before concealing them in the sterile dressing. Ensure that the catheter hub and filter are positioned comfortably for the patient and are not subject to constant pressure from lying or sitting on them.

inserting a catheter and is easy to combine with a psoas compartment block because the patient position for both techniques is the same. The posterior 'lithotomy' approach is also suitable. As both of these approaches to the sciatic nerve are at right angles to the nerve, the insulated Tuohy needle kits are recommended because they make it easier to thread the catheter in the long axis of the nerve. At the level of the popliteal fossa, both posterior and lateral approaches to the nerves can be used for inserting catheters. Use an 80 mm insulated Tuohy needle for the posterior approach because the nerves are more superficial with this approach than with the lateral approach where 100 mm Tuohy needle is necessary. In both approaches, try and identify both components (tibial and common peroneal) separately, starting with deeper tibial nerve and then withdrawing the needle slowly to locate the peroneal nerve. Inject 10–15 ml of local anaesthetic near each nerve before finally threading the catheter midway between both nerves.

Paraverterbral and psoas compartment blocks

Use the standard approaches described in Section 2, Chapter 2 (pp 54 and 79). For the thoracic paravertebral technique use a 16G Tuohy needle to locate the compartment and introduce 2–3 cm of epidural catheter into the compartment. For the psoas compartment block use a 100 or 150 mm cannula over needle, catheter through cannula technique.

Complications

The usual complications of the single-shot techniques may well occur with catheter infusions. There are additional complications that are unique to the use of continuous infusions. In particular, they must be carried out under full sterile precautions to minimise the risk of infection:

- technical difficulty and increased failure of insertion
- increased incidence of phrenic nerve paresis and Horners syndrome with brachial plexus catheters
- systemic toxicity
- vascular cannulation/haematoma
- infection
- risk of nerve damage/neuritis
- catheter problems
  - kinking
  - displacement

Injection and infusion volumes

Use normal drug concentrations and volumes to establish the block; if rapid onset is required, use lidocaine 2% and then *l*-bupivacaine or ropivacaine subsequently. The extended duration of the infusion is then achieved using either repeated bolus injections or a continuous infusion. The arguments for repeated injections or infusions are the same for both epidural and peripheral nerve catheters.

A continuous infusion via a syringe driver or a volumetric pump is easy to set up and requires less medical or nursing intervention than intermittent bolus injection but it may require larger total volumes and thus increase the risk of systemic absorption. Intermittent boluses require more intervention but allow closer control of drug usage and assessment of the pain levels. Patient-controlled infusions are well tolerated and effective. A low-volume background infusion and patient-controlled analgesia (PCA) combines both techniques satisfactorily. A 5 ml/h infusion of 0.125% *l*-bupivacaine with 2.5-ml boluses and a 30-min lock-out period gives comparable analgesia but uses less volume of solution and reduces side effects compared to a continuous infusion.

Central neuraxial blocks

Applied anatomy of the central neuraxis

Applied physiology of the spinal cord

Indications for central neuraxial blockade

Techniques of central neuraxial blocks

Introduction

There are three central neuraxial techniques in common use, each having a number of alternative names. *Spinal* (synonym: intrathecal or subarachnoid), *epidural* (extradural or peridural) and *caudal* (sacral epidural) are the preferred terms for central neuraxial anaesthesia and analgesia in this section.

The anatomy of the vertebral column, epidural space, spinal cord, dural sac and the segmental nerve roots is complex. The chapter in this text on the anatomy of the central neuraxis is limited to the core anatomical knowledge required to perform the blocks successfully and safely. For more detailed information on the relevant anatomy, the reader should consult standard anatomical reference works.

Safe and effective use of spinal, epidural and caudal blocks includes an understanding of the physiological effects that these techniques have on the cardiovascular, respiratory, gastrointestinal and genito-urinary systems. All three techniques produce similar changes in the physiological response to local anaesthetic block but the speed of onset, the extent, intensity and duration of effect will vary according to which block is used.

The techniques described in Chapter 3 for performing a spinal, epidural and caudal are standard techniques, based on conventional teaching. There are many variations and modifications of these approaches, which cannot all be accommodated in this chapter. The nature of central neuraxial blocks means that individual practitioners modify these basic techniques to suit their particular needs as they increase in confidence and experience.

Applied anatomy of the central neuraxis

The bony structures

The vertebral column provides the necessary bony strength to support the upper body weight, the flexibility to allow locomotion and protection of the spinal cord. The vertebral column consists of 24 individual vertebrae and nine fused vertebrae. The main part of the spinal column is comprised of seven cervical, 12 thoracic and five lumbar vertebrae. The five sacral and four coccygeal vertebrae are fused into two bony structures – the sacrum and the coccyx.

The vertebrae

All vertebrae have a common structure, even the fused ones. Each has an anterior *vertebral body* for strength, from which arise two *laminae* and two *pedicles* to form the *neural arch* through which the spinal cord passes. The laminae join in the posterior midline and form the spinous process. Where the pedicles and lamina meet the vertebral body, the transverse processes form lateral extensions to the vertebra. The common components of a typical vertebra are shown in Figure 3.1. Note that the structure and size of an individual vertebra varies with its particular function.

Cervical vertebrae

Cervical vertebrae have the smallest mass (as they bear little weight) and a large triangular-shaped canal to accommodate the cervical

Figure 3.1
Vertebrae: (a) Cervical, (b) Thoracic

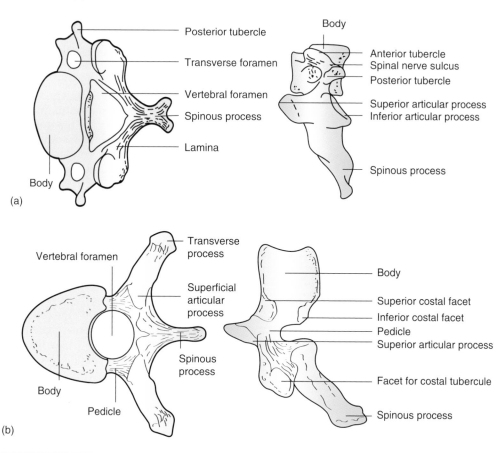

Figure 3.1 (*Continued*)
(c) lumbar

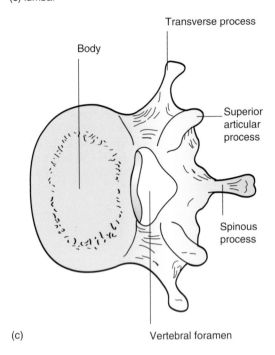

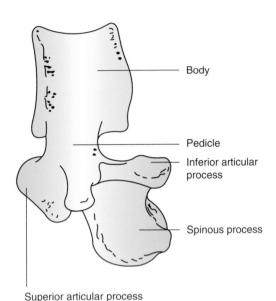

(c)   Vertebral foramen

Superior articular process

enlargement of the cord and to allow room for the cord during movement of the head and neck. The atlas (C1) and the axis (C2) have undergone highly specialised structural development to form the cranio–cervical junction. All seven cervical vertebrae have an additional component, compared to the other vertebrae – the transverse foramen within the transverse process through which the vertebral artery passes cranially.

Thoracic vertebrae

Thoracic vertebrae are characterised by progressive caudad angulation of their spinous processes as far as T7–8. The spinal canal is almost circular and they also have additional articular facets to accommodate the rib articulation.

Lumbar vertebrae

Lumbar vertebrae have the largest mass and are clearly the weight-bearing part of the column. The spinous processes are short and perpendicular as are the transverse processes. The fifth lumbar vertebra has a wedge-shaped body so that it forms an angle to articulate with the sacrum.

The spinal cord

The spinal cord has a relatively constant length of about 45 cm in the adult human despite any variation in overall body height. Similarly, the vertebral column has a relatively constant length of about 70 cm in an adult male. The cord arises as an extension of the medulla oblongata at the base of the skull and descends to terminate in the conus medullaris, the caudad tip of which generally reaches the L1/2 interspace. The exact level at which the spinal cord ends is subject to variation – between the lower border of L1 vertebral body and the lower border of L2. This reinforces the importance of performing any spinal injection at or below the L2/3 interspace to avoid inadvertent spinal cord damage.

The cord is generally cylindrical in shape (slightly flattened in the antero-posterior diameter) until it tapers into the conus medullaris but it has two enlargements at the cervical and lumbar levels where the segmental nerve supply to the upper and lower limbs leaves the cord. These two enlargements of the cord (C3–T1/2 and T9–T12) reduce the available space around the cord within the epidural space to a minimum and injections into the epidural space at these two levels should either be

Figure 3.2
Transverse section of the vertebral column and its contents at the L1 level

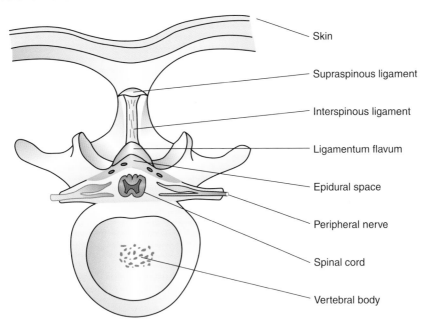

Skin

Supraspinous ligament

Interspinous ligament

Ligamentum flavum

Epidural space

Peripheral nerve

Spinal cord

Vertebral body

avoided or carried out with great caution as it may be easier to traumatise the cord at these levels than elsewhere within the vertebral column (Figure 3.2).

Blood supply to the spinal cord

This is derived primarily from the vertebral, deep cervical, intercostal and lumbar arteries. These arteries give rise to spinal branches that in turn divide into radicular feeder arteries, which accompany the segmental nerves towards the spinal cord. Beneath the pia mater, the radicular arteries anastomose to produce a longitudinal plexus from which both paired posterior spinal arteries and a single anterior spinal artery are formed. One of the lower thoracic or lumbar radicular arteries (more commonly on the left) is larger than the others and is the prime tributary vessel to the anterior spinal artery (the artery of Adamkiewicz).

The anterior spinal artery supplies the antero-lateral two thirds of the cord and the posterior arteries supply the rest of the cord. There are few, if any arterial anastomoses within the territory of the anterior spinal artery and should the vessel fail to supply the spinal cord, widespread sensory and motor loss can occur. Systemic hypotension, fat embolism,

atheromatous change, surgical damage to the artery of Adamkiewicz can all produce potentially widespread and permanent ischaemic damage to the spinal cord – the so-called 'anterior spinal artery syndrome'.

Segmental nerves

There are 31 pairs of spinal nerves (eight cervical, 12 thoracic, five lumbar, five sacral and one coccygeal) arising from the spinal cord and formed from the union of the dorsal and ventral roots. The dorsal roots are the afferent sensory input to the cord whilst the ventral roots are the efferent motor output from the cord. The anatomy of a typical segmental spinal nerve is described in Section 2, Chapter 2, p 74. The important motor effects of spinal segmental nerve blockade are shown in Figure 3.3.

Below the termination of the cord, the lumbar and sacral nerves form the *cauda equina* which offers a large surface area of nerve roots covered only by the pia mater, which accounts for the sensitivity of these nerves to local anaesthetic agents administered intrathecally.

The autonomic nervous system

The brain and spinal cord contain autonomic fibres that supply a series of ganglia with

Figure 3.3
The segmental motor supply to major muscles and joints

Upper limb			
Shoulder	C6–8	Elbow	C5–8
Wrist	C6–7	Hand	C7–T1
Trunk			
Intercostals	T1–11	Diaphragm	C3–5
Abdominal wall	T7–12		
Lower limb			
Hip flexion	L1–3	Hip extension	L5–S1
Knee flexion	L5–S1	Knee extension	L3–4
Ankle flexion	L4–5	Ankle extension	S1–2

pre-ganglionic fibres. From the ganglia, post-ganglionic fibres innervate the target organs. The sympathetic and parasympathetic systems are complementary in purpose, the combined effect being to regulate the automatic function of non-striated muscle within visceral organs and the function of a number of endocrine organs.

The sympathetic nervous system: This consists primarily of two paravertebral chains of ganglia each of which forms three cervical, 12 thoracic, five lumbar and five sacral ganglia. These ganglia have short pre-ganglionic, myelinated fibres arising within the spinal cord and emerging with the segmental nerves to form the 'white' rami communicantes. From the ganglia, unmyelinated 'grey' rami communicantes form long post-ganglionic fibres, which rejoin the ventral rami of the spinal nerves and accompany the somatic nerve supply of the target organ.

The parasympathetic nervous system: This has two separate outflows – one from the brain in the form of cranial nerve fibres (oculomotor, facial, glossopharyngeal and vagus) and the other from the spinal sacral nerves S2, 3 and 4. In contrast to the sympathetic system, the pre-ganglionic fibres are longer, the ganglia are anatomically less well defined and close to the target organs with short post-ganglionic fibres.

Central neuraxial blocks cause extensive autonomic nerve block as both the sympathetic chain and the vagal and sacral parasympathetic supply to the abdomen and pelvis are affected. Both systems are responsible for relaying visceral pain signals to the spinal cord and need to be blocked to provide analgesia to the peritoneum and the abdominal organs. Autonomic nerve blockade is also responsible for the physiological effects on the haemodynamic, gastro-intestinal

and neuroendocrine systems that accompanies central neuraxial blockade – see Section 3, Chapter 2.

The meninges

The three layers of the meninges surround the spinal cord from the foramen magnum as far down as the second sacral segment (S2). The *dura mater* is a continuation of the cerebral dura, which divides into two layers within the spinal canal. The outer layer is contiguous with the periosteum of the spinal canal whilst the inner layer forms the dura mater – a tough fibro-elastic membrane beneath which lies the delicate *arachnoid mater*. The dura mater invests the spinal cord and the spinal nerve roots forming the dural cuffs which extend laterally up to and even beyond the intervertebral foraminae. Although the arachnoid is attached to the dura there is a potential space between the layers (the sub-dural space) and inadvertent injection into this space is a recognised complication of both spinal and epidural injections. The *pia mater* is a delicate vascular layer closely adherent to the spinal cord. Lateral projections of the pia form the dentate ligaments that attach to the dura and stabilise the spinal cord. The filum terminale is the caudal extension of the pia, which anchors the spinal cord and dura to the periosteum of the coccyx.

Epidural space

The epidural space extends from the foramen magnum to the sacro-coccygeal membrane and lies between the outer surface of the dura mater and the internal bony surfaces of the spinal canal. In cross section the shape of the space is roughly triangular with the apex dorsally (posterior) but the shape and size changes at different spinal levels. In the cervical spine, the epidural space is almost oval with little room to accommodate the cervical spinal cord especially at the level of the cervical spinal enlargement. The maximum volume of the epidural space is below the level of the lumbar spinal enlargement and the end of the dural sac. The dural sac lies towards the anterior part of the epidural space and is surrounded by fat, a rich venous plexus, fewer arterial and lymphatic vessels and a number of connective tissue strands. The latter give some support to the contents of the epidural space and may, if numerous or well developed, affect the spread of local anaesthetic within the space or interfere with insertion of the epidural catheter. The paired segmental nerves cross the epidural space and exit through the intervertebral foraminae into the paravertebral space, invested in their covering of pia mater and a cuff of dura mater.

The dorsal (posterior) boundary of the epidural space is the ligamentum flavum, which is an important landmark during epidural needle insertion. It is formed from a pair of ligaments that span the intervertebral space between the laminae of adjacent vertebrae. These ligaments usually but not always bond in the midline to form a tough, yellow-coloured ligament that offers the characteristic 'woody' resistance to the passage of an epidural needle between neighbouring spinous processes and gives warning of the final approach to the epidural space. Occasionally, if the component parts of the ligament do not bond, there will be a midline gap through which the needle will pass into the epidural space without any appreciation of the usual resistance offered by the ligament.

The boundaries of the epidural space are listed in Figure 3.4.

The depth of the posterior compartment of the epidural space varies at different levels. Within the cervical spine the epidural space is only 0.5–1.0 mm deep posteriorly and may be completely absent at the C1–2 levels. Below the level of the lumbar spinal enlargement the maximum depth of the posterior compartment of the epidural space is up to 9 mm.

Figure 3.4
Boundaries of the epidural space

Superior	Fusion of the dura with the foramen magna
Inferior	Sacro-coccygeal membrane
Lateral	Vertebral pedicles and intervertebral foraminae
Anterior	Posterior longitudinal ligament and vertebral bodies
Posterior	Vertebral laminae and ligamentum flavum

Caudal anatomy

The sacrum is formed from the fusion of the five sacral vertebrae into a shield-like structure whose function is to provide a strong, weight-bearing joint between the pelvis and the vertebral column. The normal anatomy of the sacrum is subject to great variation in the extent to which the laminae of the five sacral vertebrae fuse in the midline to form the sacral canal. The sacral hiatus normally results from the failure of the lamina of S4 and 5 to fuse but it can vary in size from complete absence (approximately 5% of the population) to complete bifida of the sacrum. Within the sacral canal, the dural sac ends at the S2 level in adults, a level which approximates to a line drawn between the posterior superior iliac spines. The sacral nerves leave the sacral canal through the anterior sacral foraminae to form the sacral plexus within the pelvis and the dorsal sensory nerves exit via the posterior foraminae to supply the skin over the sacrum and natal cleft.

Applied physiology of the spinal cord

Cerebrospinal fluid

Cerebrospinal fluid (CSF) is a clear fluid with a mean specific gravity of 1.006 at 37°C, which is actively secreted by the choroid plexii in the lateral and fourth ventricles at a rate of up to 500 ml per day. There is no active flow, movement occurring by diffusion and changes in posture. Absorption occurs (at equilibrium with production) via the arachnoid villi of the major cerebral sinuses. The typical composition of CSF is shown in Figure 3.5.

Spinal anaesthesia

A small volume of local anaesthetic agent is injected directly into the CSF to produce spinal anaesthesia. The local is usually injected in the lumbar region below the level of L1/2, where the spinal cord ends. The mixing of the injected fluid within the CSF is a matter of both simple diffusion and bulk movement of the fluid, which has different physico-chemical properties to CSF. A number of factors affect the spread of local anaesthetic within the CSF; these are listed in Figure 3.6.

The posture of the patient during and immediately after the injection and the density of the local anaesthetic solution are the two most important influences on the duration, maximal spread and quality of the block. The ratio of the density of the solution to that of CSF is expressed as baricity (where isobaricity equals 1.0). If the injection is made at the L3/4 interspace with the patient in the left lateral position and the patient is then immediately turned supine, hypo- and hyperbaric solutions produce different effects due to their distribution patterns.

Hypobaric solutions are not commonly available in the UK now but have been used traditionally for lower abdominal and lower extremity surgery, as they tend to be restricted to the top of the lumbar lordosis when the patient lies supine. With the use of head-up tilt, the height of the block can be encouraged in a cephalad direction but at the expense of a patchy quality of anaesthesia and an unpredictable height. Head-down tilt will restrict the caudad limit of the block.

Isobaric solutions are not influenced by posture and may be expected to produce a block influenced more by level of injection and volume. Commercially produced bupivacaine (normally described as isobaric) is slightly hypobaric (0.999) at body temperature and can produce unpredictable results with changing posture.

Hyperbaric bupivacaine (0.5% bupivacaine in 8% glucose) is the most commonly used drug for spinal anaesthesia in the UK at present. As hyperbaric solutions are hypertonic they remain affected by posture for up to 30 min after injection and so sensory levels may change within that time. This explains why so-called saddle blocks and unilateral spinals can rarely, if ever, be achieved with hyperbaric solutions.

The effects of a spinal anaesthetic on the physiology of the major organ systems are related primarily to the height of the block. Specific organ systems affected are detailed below.

Figure 3.5
Composition of CSF

Total volume (brain and spinal cord)	~130 ml
Volume around spinal cord	~35 ml
CSF pressure in lumbar region	60–100 mmH$_2$O (lateral)
	200–250 mmH$_2$O (sitting)
Hydrogen ion concentration	40–45 nmol/l
Protein content	20–40 mg/l
Specific gravity	1006

Figure 3.6
Factors influencing intrathecal spread of solution

Major influence	Minor influence
• Baricity of solution	• Intervertebral level of injection
• Posture of patient	• Height of patient
• Volume of solution	• Age of patient
• Mass of drug injected	• Weight of patient
• Volume of CSF	• Speed of injection
	• Induced turbulence (barbotage)
	• Posture

Nervous system

The intensity of neural blockade is greatest at the level at which the needle is inserted into the spinal canal. Under the influence of posture and gravity, there is usually complete neural blockade caudad to the injection site whilst cephalad to it the concentration of local anaesthetic decreases, producing a differential nerve block of the sensory, motor and autonomic fibres. Sympathetic fibres are most sensitive and may be blocked 2–6 segments higher than sensory fibres, which in turn may be a few segments higher than the associated motor block.

Respiratory system

Below the thoracic nerves, spinal anaesthesia has no clinical effect on respiratory function but as the intercostal nerves become progressively blocked, active expiratory mechanics are impaired producing a reduction in vital capacity and expiratory reserve volume. Tidal volume and other inspiratory mechanics remain normal due to increased diaphragmatic movement. Patients may complain of dyspnoea and may lose the ability to cough effectively. If there is exceptional cephalad spread and the cervical nerves become affected, apnoea due to phrenic nerve blockade can occur.

Cardiovascular system

Progressive blockade of the thoraco-lumbar sympathetic outflow produces increasing vasodilatation of the resistance and capacitance vessels and a reduction of 15–18% in systemic vascular resistance. If the cardiac output is maintained, there will be a similar fall in mean arterial pressure. If, however, the cardiac output falls due to a reduction in preload (for example due to hypovolaemia or a reduction in venous return due to postural changes) then hypotension may develop rapidly especially if the block reaches the cardioaccelerator fibres above the level of T4/5 when a reflex bradycardia may occur. Above the level of the block there is usually compensatory vasoconstriction but this is not sufficient to prevent significant falls in arterial pressure if the block is extensive.

Gastro-intestinal system

Sympathetic blockade allows vagal, parasympathetic activity to predominate. Gastric emptying and peristalsis continue, sphincters relax and the bowel is generally contracted. This may preclude the use of central blockade in patients with obstructed bowel, at least until the obstruction has been relieved. However, the incidence of post-operative ileus is reduced by spinal and epidural blockade and this is one of their main benefits. Nausea and vomiting can occur as a result of the unopposed vagal activity, if the peritoneal contents are stimulated in the conscious patient.

Epidural anaesthesia

The effects of epidural anaesthesia on the major organ systems are similar to those of spinal anaesthesia with the height of the block being the major determinant. In a patient with compromised cardiovascular or respiratory reserve, the slower onset of epidural blockade gives more time to manage the onset of hypotension and other side effects, although against this advantage must be weighed the risks of the need for a much larger dose of local anaesthetic drug. The spread of local anaesthetic solution within the epidural space and thus the

Figure 3.7
Factors affecting spread of epidural solutions

Factors	Comment
Drug mass	Drug mass is critical and more important than either volume or concentration.
Drug volume	For a given drug mass, larger volume gives more spread than a small volume.
Site of injection	The epidural space increases in volume in the cervico-caudad direction. Thus a given volume will produce greater spread in the cervical > thoracic > lumbar > sacral. Onset is fastest and the block most intense in the dermatomes nearest the site of injection.
Age	A given volume spreads further with increasing age over 40 years.
Raised abdominal pressure	Smaller volumes may be needed in pregnancy and morbid obesity.
Patient position	Prolonged sitting position may reduce upward spread. Earlier onset of block in dependant side in lateral position.
Injection technique	Slow 'unfractionated' injection of dose through needle gives more complete symmetrical blocks than 'fractionated' or incremental doses via catheter.

ultimate height of block is determined by a number of factors (Figure 3.7).

Caudal anaesthesia

The effect of caudal anaesthesia is limited to the lumbar and sacral nerves and therefore there will be less effect on cardiovascular, respiratory and gastro-intestinal performance than other epidural techniques. Motor weakness is limited to the legs and sensory loss is usually sub-umbilical. Autonomic disturbance is limited to bladder and anorectal dysfunction as both sympathetic and pelvic parasympathetic outflow is blocked.

Indications for central neuraxial blockade

Spinal

Spinal anaesthesia is used for a wide variety of both elective and emergency surgical procedures below the level of the umbilicus. It is customary to use a spinal as the sole anaesthetic technique, supplemented by light intravenous or oral sedation if appropriate. A spinal block can be combined with a general anaesthetic if the circumstances are such that the benefits of such a combination are worthwhile but this is not a common practice. Owing to the relatively short duration of a spinal anaesthetic, post-operative analgesia is brief and requires additional treatment with suitable drugs. For surgery above the umbilicus, high spinals are now rarely used because of associated difficulties of maintaining spontaneous ventilation and abolishing the painful stimuli from traction on the peritoneum and pressure on the diaphragm.

Epidural

An epidural can be used as the sole anaesthetic technique for surgery within the abdomen and on the lower limbs but it is more usual to combine epidural anaesthesia with a light general anaesthetic. Epidural infusions are extensively used for acute and chronic pain relief (Figure 3.8).

Caudal

Indications

There are multiple indications for the use of caudal anaesthesia, listed in Figure 3.9. Most caudal injections are single-shot injections, although it is possible to insert an epidural catheter into the sacral canal and use it for prolonged infusions, in the same way as lumbar or thoracic infusions are used. This is the preferred route of catheter insertion for paediatric epidural infusions in babies and small children; although it is a potentially infected area and precautions against sepsis must be rigorously maintained.

Spinal or epidural?

It can be difficult to decide between the relative merits of a spinal or an epidural when assessing

Figure 3.8
Indications for epidural anaesthesia and analgesia

Surgery
- Thoracic
  - pulmonary
  - cardiac
  - vascular
- Abdominal
  - gastro-intestinal
  - gynaecological
  - urological
- Lower extremity
  - orthopaedic and trauma

Acute pain relief
- Post-operative analgesia
- Trauma
  - rib fractures
  - pelvic and lower extremity injuries
- Miscellaneous
  - pancreatitis
  - ischaemic limb pain

Chronic pain states
- Chronic benign pain
- Cancer pain

Figure 3.9
Indications for caudal anaesthesia

Adult
- Surgery
  - anorectal
  - gynaecology
  - orthopaedic surgery
- Obstetric
  - episiotomy
  - removal of placenta
- Chronic pain
  - coccydynia
  - spinal manipulation

Paediatric
- Major abdominal and orthopaedic surgery
- Inguinal hernia repair
- Surgery to genitalia

a particular patient for the most appropriate anaesthetic technique. The significant differences between spinal and epidural approaches are summarised in Figure 3.10.

Figure 3.10
Differences between spinal and epidural techniques

	Spinal	Epidural
Onset	2–5 min	20–30 min
Duration	2–3 h (single shot)	3–5 h
Drug volume	2.5–4 ml	20–30 ml
Quality of block	Rapid surgical anaesthesia motor = sensory	May be inadequate in some dermatomes sensory may be > motor

The above differences apply to single-shot, local anaesthetic blocks and the addition of adjuvant drugs (such as opioids or α-2 agonists) can alter the characteristics of each technique. With regard to the epidural route it is customary to insert a catheter to allow top-up doses or prolonged infusions whereas spinal catheters are only now becoming popular and are not yet commonplace. Combined spinal and epidural (CSE) anaesthesia is increasingly used, especially for obstetric surgery in order to utilise the benefits of both techniques. Surgical block can be rapidly established with a small dose of spinal bupivacaine (2–2.5 ml of hyperbaric solution) followed by the slower onset of a low dose epidural which can be used to extend operating time and post-operative analgesia.

In summary, spinals provide rapid onset, short duration surgical anaesthesia below the umbilicus with small doses of drug. Epidurals have a slower onset time, require large doses of drug and produce less dense surgical anaesthesia but can be used more flexibly in the lumbar and thoracic regions and their duration may be extended for days or weeks for analgesia by the insertion of a catheter.

Techniques of central neuraxial blocks

Introduction

The majority of epidural injections involve the insertion of an epidural catheter whereas, traditionally, spinal anaesthesia has been restricted to single-shot injection. Epidural catheter infusions are used extensively following major thoraco-abdominal surgery and continuous spinal techniques are increasingly being used for some high-risk surgical cases – especially in vascular and orthopaedic surgery to provide both surgical anaesthesia and post-operative analgesia for lower abdominal and lower limb surgery.

Similarly, although the majority of caudal injections are single-shot, continuous caudal catheter infusions are used in paediatric surgery for major lower abdominal and lower limb procedures.

Spinal anaesthesia

Equipment

Spinal anaesthesia requires specialised needles and introducers in addition to the general equipment necessary for central nerve blocks (Figure 3.11). There is an inevitable incidence of post-dural puncture headache (PDPH) with spinal anaesthesia ranging from 0.2% to 24% and many designs of needle have been introduced to try and reduce this problem. Currently the lowest incidence of PDPH is associated with very narrow gauge, short bevel needles (26–29G) and 24G pencil point, Whitacre tip designs or the more specialised designs with a large side-opening hole. The narrow gauge and relatively blunt tips of these needles require insertion through a properly designed introducer, which should be closely matched to the type of spinal needle being used to avoid tip damage.

Although pencil point needles may have a lower risk for PDPH, there may be a slightly increased risk of spinal cord or nerve root injury with the use of these needle designs. The blunt tip and the variable distance of the lateral orifice behind the tip mean that the needle needs more force to insert it through the dura and it may need to be inserted deeper into the intrathecal space for the orifice to fully penetrate the dura.

Technique

Spinal anaesthesia should be carried out as a strictly aseptic procedure. Carry out a full surgical scrub of the hands and forearms and wear a surgical cap, gown and sterile gloves. Sterilise the patient's lumbar skin with a suitable antiseptic solution and use sterile surgical drapes to prepare an appropriate area of the back for the spinal injection.

Successful spinal anaesthesia depends on a reliable lumbar puncture technique. First establish venous access with a wide bore cannula and then position the patient either in the *lateral* position with the spine flexed maximally to open up the gaps between the vertebral spines or in the *sitting* position with the feet placed on a low stool at the side of the bed and the elbows resting on the thighs (Figure 3.12). Each position has drawbacks and

Figure 3.11
Tip design of spinal needles. (a) Euro pencil point, (b) lancet point and (c) pencil point (reproduced with the kind permission of Smiths Medical)

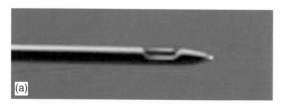
(a)

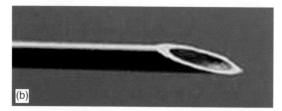
(b)

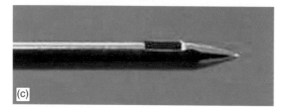
(c)

Figure 3.12
Patient positions (a) sitting and (b) lateral for spinal anaesthesia

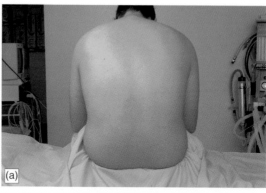
(a)

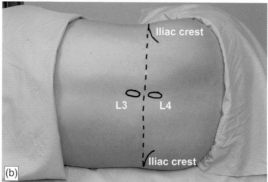
(b)

advantages and the choice is usually made on personal preference. In either case, a skilled assistant is necessary to position the patient correctly, maintain and support the posture and establish a rapport with them during the conduct of the block.

A line joining both iliac crests (the intercristal or Tuffier's line) passes across the spine of L4 and is a reliable landmark for locating the L3/4 interspace which is usually easily defined and is the one most often used. The technique for spinal anaesthesia is described below (Figure 3.13):

- Sterilise the skin over the lumbar spine with a spirit-based antiseptic and raise a skin wheal with 1% lidocaine over the appropriate interspace. Inject a further 2–3 ml of lidocaine into the subcutaneous tissue.
- Anchor the skin over the interspace by pressing the non-dominant index finger on the spine of the cephalad vertebra and insert the needle or introducer in the midline at 90° to the skin (a,b). Feedback from the needle tip will indicate progress of the needle through the supraspinous and interspinous ligaments,

the ligamentum flavum and sometimes the dura mater. If bone is contacted, withdraw the needle to the subcutaneous tissue and re-direct the introducer and/or the needle slightly cephalad in the first instance.
- Puncture of the dura is usually obvious and when the stylet is removed cerebrospinal fluid (CSF) should flow freely (c).

Note that 22G needles are robust enough to be used without an introducer in patients with calcified ligaments or other anatomical difficulties and are recommended for elderly patients where these problems are more common and the risk of PDPH is very low. If an introducer is required, it should be inserted into the deep layers of the interspinous ligament, so that the needle has only a short distance to travel. Narrow gauge needles may be deviated or damaged by the ligamentum flavum, calcified ligaments or osteophytes and also will give little feedback. After performing the block the blood pressure, pulse rate and electro-cardiograph (ECG) should be monitored, as the onset of sympathetic nerve blockade is quite

Figure 3.13
Technique of spinal anaesthesia (lateral position)

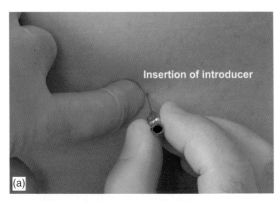
(a) Insertion of introducer

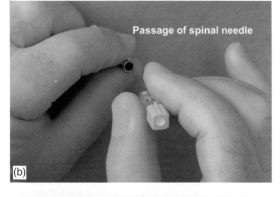
(b) Passage of spinal needle

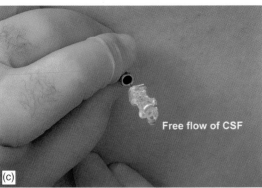
(c) Free flow of CSF

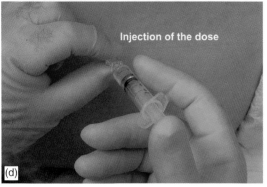
(d) Injection of the dose

rapid. When using 3 ml of 0.5% bupivacaine in 8% glucose (hyperbaric solution) (d), motor and sensory loss will be apparent within a few minutes but the block may not be fully complete for up to 25 min. Sensory block can be tested using a blunt pinprick or loss of temperature sensation with an alcohol swab. Dermatomes should be tested bilaterally starting in the dermatome nearest to the level of injection. Motor loss is usually estimated using the Bromage scale or a similar objective scale of effect (Figure 3.14).

Normally, the whole procedure is conducted with the patient conscious or lightly premedicated, so as to maintain verbal contact and co-operation. If turning the patient is likely to be painful (for example those with fractured neck of femur), intravenous ketamine 0.5 mg/kg may be administered to provide analgesia during insertion of the spinal.

Continuous spinal anaesthesia

A 19G Tuohy needle is used to puncture the dura using the same technique as for a single-shot spinal technique. Once CSF is identified, a narrow gauge (larger than 24G) epidural catheter is introduced via the needle into the CSF. Only 3 cm is introduced and aimed in a cephalad direction to minimise the risk of neurological damage previously described with continuous spinal anaesthesia (CSA) when microcatheters (25G or smaller) were used. Despite the large hole made in the dura by the needle, the incidence of PDPH in a non-obstetric population is estimated to be about 1%.

The major advantage of CSA is that it allows incremental doses to be used to produce rapid onset spinal anaesthesia with cardiovascular stability which can then be modified by further small doses to produce a predictable and dense blockade for surgery and then used for post-operative analgesia for up to 24 h. CSA has been used for periods of longer than 24 h but experience is limited and data on the safety of prolonged infusions is sparse.

Drugs, doses and volumes

Single-dose spinal blockade

The volume of local anaesthetic required to produce spinal anaesthesia varies according to the dermatomal spread required. Figure 3.15 gives a guide to drug administration for various operative sites.

Figure 3.14
The Bromage motor block scale

THE BROMAGE MOTOR BLOCK SCALE (1965)		
Degree of motor block	Bromage criterion	% score
1. No block	Full flexion of knees and feet	0
2. Partial block	Just able to flex knees plus full flexion of feet	33
3. Almost complete	Unable to flex knees, some foot flexion still	66
4. Complete	Unable to move legs or feet	100

Figure 3.15
Drug doses in spinal anaesthesia

Operation site	Block level	Drug volume (hyperbaric bupivacaine 0.5%) (ml)
Perianal	L4/5	2.5
Lower limb	L1/2	2.75–3.0
Urogenital	T10	2.75–3.0
Lower abdominal	T6/7	3.0–3.25

Hyperbaric bupivacaine 0.5% gives a reliable surgical block for 2–3 h. The above doses apply to a fit adult of normal stature (70 kg) and smaller volumes may be necessary for higher-risk patients. Plain 'isobaric' bupivacaine 0.5% 3–4 ml is also commonly used but is less reliable above T10. Lidocaine 5% in 8% glucose is sometimes indicated for short duration blocks; 2.5–3.0 ml lasts up to 1 h at T10 and up to 2 h in the lower limbs.

Continuous spinal blockade

Increments of 0.5% isobaric bupivacaine are administered in 0.5 ml volumes to a maximum of 3 ml until the desired height and density of blockade are achieved.

Complications

Some complications (hypotension, urinary retention and bradycardia) are actually physiological consequences of central neural blockade and should not represent a clinical problem if correctly managed. If management is inappropriate, secondary effects such as nausea and vomiting, faintness or vasovagal loss of consciousness may follow.

Headache

Loss of CSF through the dural puncture site will produce a low-pressure headache due to traction on the cranial meninges. The main characteristics of a spinal headache are that it is minimal when lying flat, is severe when sitting or standing, occurs in the occipital and bi-frontal distribution and may be worsened by coughing or straining. In severe cases the traction may produce cranial nerve symptoms with alterations in vision and hearing. Onset is usually within 24 h of the injection and the majority of PDPH's diminish rapidly with rest, oral analgesia and adequate hydration and should resolve within 7 days.

Occasionally, more invasive treatment is required in high-risk groups such as pregnant women and after puncture with large bore needles. An *epidural blood patch*, in which 20–30 ml of the patient's own blood is withdrawn from a vein under the strictest sterile precautions and injected through an epidural needle placed as close to the level of the dural puncture as possible, is very effective at relieving a PDPH with over 90% success with the first injection. Other causes of headache should be considered before ascribing the cause to the spinal and a careful history of events should be elicited as headaches are a very frequent complaint after surgery.

Neurological sequelae

Temporary symptoms of paraesthesia, hypoanaesthesia and motor weakness may follow spinal anaesthesia but are not necessarily the result of trauma to a spinal nerve root. These symptoms occur from pressure, surgical trauma or stretching of the root or peripheral nerve and the great majority resolve spontaneously within a few weeks. Serious, permanent neurological damage is extremely rare (less than 1:10,000) but in view of the serious consequences of such an event, any neurological sequelae should be formally examined by a neurologist with experience of this type of damage as soon as the problem arises. Other rare causes of neurological damage include brain damage and anterior spinal artery syndrome due to excessive and prolonged hypotension, infection (meningitis and epidural abscess), arachnoiditis and cauda equina syndrome (both associated with the injection of incorrect solutions) and are usually the result of a failure of technique.

Commonly, but not invariably, the subsequent development of temporary and permanent nerve damage is associated with pain on needle insertion or drug injection. It is important that the patient is able to communicate effectively with the anaesthetist during the block performance so that any painful stimuli can be reported. Sedation should be limited so that communication is still possible and general anaesthesia (if required) should be induced after the spinal injection is complete.

Localised pain due to the needle passing through the various tissue layers is relatively common and can be alleviated by injecting lidocaine into the area before commencing the needle insertion. Pain caused by the spinal needle touching the spinal cord or nerve roots is quite distinct and is typically described as a painful 'electric shock' down one or both legs, although it may be localised to the lumbar and buttock area. If the patient complains of this type of sensation, stop the procedure immediately, remove the needle and consider whether to continue with the spinal or change to a different anaesthetic technique. On no account should the patient's complaints of pain be disregarded.

Epidural anaesthesia

Equipment

In addition to the general equipment necessary for regional anaesthesia (see previously) a suitable epidural pack will be required. Packs containing sterile, single use, disposable equipment; a loss of resistance syringe, Tuohy needle, catheter and bacterial filter are widely available. There is no longer a place for re-usable equipment of this type.

Technique

The same sterile precautions outlined above for the spinal block are required for an epidural technique, especially as an indwelling epidural catheter will increase the risk of infection for the duration of its placement. The practical technique of lumbar midline approach to the epidural space is described below (Figure 3.16):

- the Tuohy needle, the loss of resistance syringe, the catheter and filter must be examined and prepared for use

- connect the filter and catheter and fill with saline to ensure free passage of solution
- position the patient in either the lateral or sitting position as for a spinal injection and identify the appropriate vertebral interspace
- sterilise and drape the area, raise a skin wheal with 1% lignocaine and anchor the skin over the cephalad spine of the interspace with the non-dominant index finger
- insert a 21G hypodermic needle at right angles to the skin exactly in the midline of the interspace to inject more local anaesthetic into the interspinous ligaments and identify the route of the Tuohy needle
- insert the Tuohy needle in the direction indicated by the hypodermic needle. The needle will pass easily through the superficial layers but as it passes through the supraspinous and interspinous ligaments, resistance will become more obvious. If the needle strikes bone withdraw it slightly and re-angle slightly cephalad but still in the midline. Once the needle is located in the deeper layers of the interspinous ligament,

Figure 3.16
Technique for epidural insertion (lateral position)

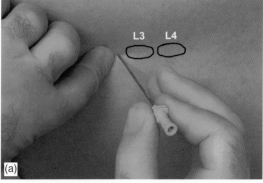

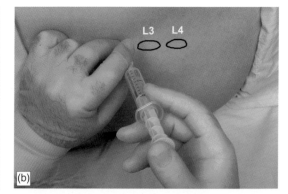

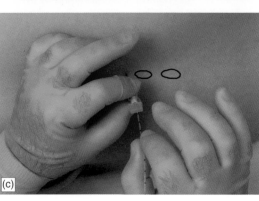

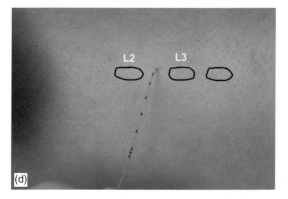

remove the trochar and attach the loss of resistance syringe filled with air or saline as required

- carefully advance the needle and syringe combination through the deep layers of the interspinous ligament and into the ligamentum flavum
- constantly check for loss of resistance as the needle is advanced through the ligament, which is 3–5 mm thick in the midline

Using air to detect loss of resistance

Advance the needle in 1–2 mm increments, frequently stopping to check the loss of resistance syringe with light bounces of the plunger with the thumb of the dominant hand. If using a two-handed technique, hold the wings of the Tuohy needle with the thumb and forefinger of each hand, bracing the hands against the skin of the back.

After advancing 1–2 mm, stabilise the needle with the non-dominant hand and use the dominant hand to test for loss of resistance, repeating the process until loss of resistance is identified. If using a single-handed technique, brace the non-dominant hand against the skin to stabilise and control forward movement of the syringe/needle combination.

Advance the combination with the dominant hand, intermittently stopping to test for loss of resistance.

Using saline to detect loss of resistance

Advance the needle slowly and continually with the dominant hand, maintaining constant pressure on the plunger of the loss of resistance syringe.

Brace the non-dominant hand against the skin of the back to stabilise the needle/syringe combination and control forward progress. As the tip of the needle enters the epidural space, there will be a simultaneous loss of resistance in the syringe, sometimes an audible 'click' and a tactile feeling of the needle advancing more easily. Immediately control further needle advancement within the epidural space.

Immobilise the Tuohy needle once the loss of resistance occurs, carefully remove the syringe and check that no blood or CSF drains from the needle. CSF will normally emerge from a Tuohy needle with sufficient volume and velocity to leave no doubt as to its identity, even if saline has been used to detect loss of resistance!

Figure 3.17
Loss of resistance (LOR) to air or saline?

Air	Saline
Requires LOR syringe	Ordinary syringe
Intermittent testing and movement of needle	Continuous pressure on plunger and movement of needle
Easy to learn	More difficult to learn
One- or two-handed control of needle	One-handed control only
Air bubbles may form in space and expand with N_2O	Saline may be confused with CSF

There are advocates for the use of both air and saline for detecting entry into the epidural space and each technique has its own benefits and drawbacks. These are summarised in Figure 3.17.

Only 3 ml of air or saline (or less) should be injected in order to minimise bubble formation, dilution of local anaesthetic and confusion with CSF. In distinguishing saline from CSF, saline should be cold on the skin compared to CSF and CSF will show positive for glucose on proprietary stick testing.

Inserting the catheter

Once the epidural space is identified, calculate the depth of the epidural space from the skin.

Count the number of visible 1 cm markers on the shaft of the needle and subtract that number from 8 cm, which is the total length of a standard Tuohy epidural needle shaft (not including the plastic or metal hub). The catheter needs to be inserted about 4–5 cm into the epidural space. Less than 4 cm may increase the risk of the catheter being dislodged by patient movement and greater than 5–6 cm increases the risks of the catheter emigrating from the epidural space out through an intervertebral foramen, into the CSF or subdural space or becoming knotted within the epidural space. Most commercially available catheters are graduated in 10 cm lengths with the distal 10 cm marked at 1 cm intervals.

Insert the catheter through the Tuohy needle into the epidural space, noting the depth of insertion by counting the markers on the catheter. The catheter may need some firm pressure to enter the space after which it should continue to enter the space freely. If the catheter will not advance despite firm 'persuasion', remove it gently from the needle and re-confirm needle position within the epidural space using the loss of resistance syringe. If the catheter becomes stuck after initial entry, do not withdraw the catheter through the needle as this may result in the tip of the catheter shearing off and remaining in the epidural space. Remove both the needle and the catheter together and begin the process again.

It is normal practice to insert the catheter until the 15 or 20 cm marker reaches the end of the hub, depending on the exact depth of the epidural space from the skin.

Carefully withdraw the needle from the epidural space, ensuring that the catheter is not accidentally withdrawn with the needle. When the needle has been removed, gently withdraw the catheter until the desired depth marker is just visible at the skin puncture site.

Check that no blood or CSF runs back up the catheter by lowering it below the level of the spine and then raising it above the level of the spine, observing a free movement of the saline meniscus in the catheter.

Re-attach the catheter hub and filter and apply a sterile dressing to the epidural catheter site, ensuring that the catheter is securely attached to the skin of the back and over a shoulder so that the filter and hub can be secured to the anterior chest wall.

Drugs, doses and volumes

Single-shot technique

A test dose through the needle of 3 ml of 2% lidocaine plus epinephrine 1:200,000 may detect inadvertent spinal or intravascular injection, denoted by the rapid onset of a spinal block or a sudden tachycardia (although there is an incidence of false negative test doses). The local anaesthetic agent may be injected slowly over 2 min in 5 ml aliquots to allow for detection of signs of impending toxicity.

Catheter techniques

The initial dose of local anaesthetic agent may be administered through the needle followed by insertion of a catheter for subsequent top up doses. This method dilates the epidural space, allows easier insertion of the catheter, and produces a more rapid onset of anaesthesia and fewer missed segments. Alternatively, the catheter is inserted immediately loss of

Figure 3.18
Drug doses in epidural anaesthesia

Block height	Drug (volume)	Duration (h)
Lumbosacral (L1–S5 approximately)	lidocaine 2% (20–25 ml)	2–3
	bupivacaine 0.5% (15–20 ml)	4–6
	ropivacaine 0.75% (15–20 ml)	4–6
Thoraco-lumbar (T5–L4/5 approximately)	lidocaine 2% (25–30 ml)	2–3
	bupivacaine 0.5% (15–20 ml)	4–6
	ropivacaine 0.75% (15–20 ml)	4–6

resistance is confirmed, the test dose administered and the main dose given in incremental doses via the catheter. Figure 3.18 shows some indicative dosing requirements for a fit adult male with the injection made at L3/4. Lidocaine is usually used with 1:200,000 epinephrine to reduce absorption and prolong duration. Bupivacaine 0.5% offers the same duration and quality of sensory block as ropivacaine 0.5% but gives a better quality motor block.

Whichever method of epidural injection is used, the ECG, heart rate, oxygen saturation and blood pressure must be monitored frequently as the block develops over 15–20 min. The development of segmental sensory loss should be monitored by testing of dermatomal levels and motor block monitored by using the Bromage scoring system as for a spinal block.

Complications

Complications of epidural block are similar to those of a spinal block but there is a difference of severity and incidence for each of the following complications.

PDPH

If the dura is accidentally punctured, there is a higher risk of headache developing and the headache is more severe than with a spinal PDPH due to the larger hole made in the dura. In non-obstetric patients about half of the patients who have a dural puncture will develop a headache severe enough to require a blood patch but in the obstetric population over 90% of sufferers will require one.

Figure 3.19
Causes of back pain after epidural or spinal block

Cause	Notes
Needle track pain	Localised and temporary
Postural or labour	Extremes of posture during surgery or labour
Drug or additive	2-Chloroprocaine and EDTA
Epidural abscess	Rare but important to diagnose and treat early
Epidural haematoma	Rare but important to diagnose and treat early
Recurrence of previous low back pain	

Back pain

Back pain is sometimes reported after epidural (and spinal) anaesthesia and may be related to several causes (Figure 3.19).

Epidural abscess

This rare but dangerous problem can result in permanent neurological damage unless recognised and treated aggressively by removal of catheter, intravenous antibiotics, urgent radiological scanning and surgical evacuation if necessary. It may arise spontaneously or track along epidural catheters and has been reported

Figure 3.20
Guidelines for the use of central blocks in patients with disordered clotting mechanisms

- International normalised ratio (INR) less than 1.5
- Platelet count in excess of 90,000/mm^3
- Bleeding time less than 16 min
- Partial thromboplastin time not prolonged
- Prothrombin time not more than 2 s over control

after epidural blood patching in bacteraemic patients.

Epidural haematoma

Although reported after diagnostic lumbar puncture, haematoma formation is very rare after spinal and epidural anaesthesia. The majority of reported cases occur in patients with a coagulopathy or on anticoagulant treatment. Current knowledge suggests that it is safe to use spinal and epidural techniques in patients receiving prophylactic heparinisation for surgery if appropriate guidelines are followed (Section 1, p 12). If there is any doubt, then the following limits (Figure 3.20) may help to decide if it is safe to proceed with a central block. The same criteria apply to removing as well as inserting an epidural catheter.

Caudal anaesthesia

In pre-adolescent children, there is a predictable relationship between age, volume of injection and height of block but pubertal growth changes the volume and shape of the sacral canal and this relationship is lost in adults.

Equipment

A 22G short bevel needle should be used for adults and larger children and a 23G hypodermic needle for smaller children and babies. For prolonged anaesthesia and post-operative analgesia in children, continuous caudal epidurals, employing a 20G epidural catheter inserted through an 18G Tuohy needle, are becoming popular.

Technique (Figure 3.21)

It is most common to administer a caudal after inducing general anaesthesia. As with other central neuraxial techniques, strict asepsis is necessary when performing a caudal block. The practical technique is described below:

- Place the patient in the lateral position as for a spinal or lumbar epidural. Note that the posterior superior iliac spines and the sacral hiatus form an equilateral triangle (a).
- Use the index finger of the non-dominant hand to palpate the sacral cornuae either side of the hiatus which normally feels like a small depression between the bony landmarks (b).
- With the hiatus located, sterilise and prepare the area and insert the needle at an angle of about 60° to the skin through the subcutaneous tissues. The sacro-coccygeal membrane is tough and offers obvious resistance to the needle (c).
- Once through the membrane, re-angle the needle to 20–30° (Figure 3.21) and carefully advance the needle only 1–2 mm, ensuring that it remains in free space. If it strikes bone or will not advance freely, withdraw slightly and re-position the needle or begin the whole procedure again (d).

Figure 3.21
Technique for caudal anaesthesia

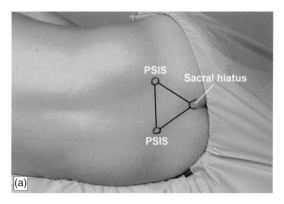

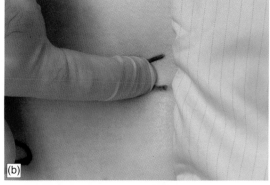

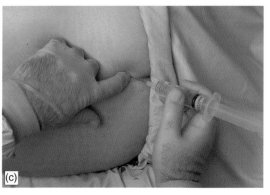

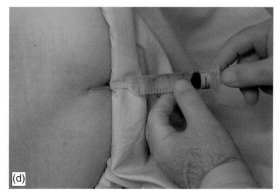

Figure 3.22
Drug doses for paediatric caudal block (0.25% bupivacaine)

Block height	Volume (ml/kg)
Lumbosacral	0.5
Thoracolumbar	1.0
Mid-thoracic	1.25

- Do not advance the needle more than 1–2 mm within the sacral canal, especially in children, because the dural sac extends beyond S2 in some individuals.
- Aspirate to check for blood and CSF and then slowly inject 3 ml of chosen solution to test for low resistance to injection. If this feels normal and there is no subcutaneous swelling denoting needle misplacement in the superficial tissues, slowly inject the main dose, with frequent aspiration checks.

Drugs, doses and volumes

Paediatric

The linear relationship between age, volume and segmental spread is utilised in a number of formulae. One of the best known is that of Armitage (1979) and this is shown in Figure 3.22.

If the volume of bupivacaine used exceeds 20 ml, motor blockade can be minimised by using 0.19% bupivacaine (dilute three parts bupivacaine with one part normal saline) and use the full calculated volume as above. Lidocaine 1% in the same volumes gives analgesia for 3–4 h compared to 6–8 h for bupivacaine.

Adults

The 25–30 ml of 0.5% bupivacaine provides 6–8 h of sub-umbilical analgesia with a variable degree of segmental spread and motor blockade. If analgesia is necessary only within the sacral nerves, 20 ml is sufficient.

Complications

Incorrect needle placement

Incorrect needle placement is the commonest problem of the technique and is usually a matter of difficulty palpating landmarks. If the needle is too superficial, then the only adverse effect is a subcutaneous injection and a failed block. If the needle is inserted too deeply, it can pass through the sacro-coccygeal joint into the pelvic cavity and thus the viscera, risking contamination of the epidural space. In pregnant patients, there are reports of the needle entering the birth canal and damaging the fetal head.

Intravascular injection

Intravascular injection is a risk due to the rich plexus of veins within the sacral canal. If the marrow of the sacral vertebra is cannulated and the dose injected, rapid systemic absorption can occur.

Infection

Infection from a dirty technique in a potentially unsterile area is a constant risk.

Dural puncture

Dural puncture is an uncommon but important complication because of the potentially large volume of local anaesthetic solution that can be inadvertently injected intrathecally.

Section 4

Appendix

Abbreviations

Further reading

Abbreviations

ACT	Activated clotting time
ADH	Antidiuretic hormone
Adren	Adrenaline
AIDS	Acquired immune deficiency syndrome
Alpha-2	Alpha-2 adrenergic receptor
APTT	Activated partial thromboplastin time
ASIS	Anterior superior iliac spine
ATP	Adenosine triphosphate
bupiv	bupivacaine
C	Cervical (nerve root or dermatome)
cm	Centimetre
CN	Cranial nerve
CNS	Central nervous system
Concn	Concentration
CPR	Cardiopulmonary resuscitation
CSF	Cerebrospinal fluid
CT	Computerised (axial) tomography
CVA	Cerebrovascular accident
CVS	Cardiovascular system
Dur	Duration
ECG	Electrocardiogram
EMLA	Eutectic mixture of local anaesthetics
ENT	Ear nose and throat
ESRA	European Society of Regional Anaesthesia
G (SWG)	Steel wire gauge
h	Hour
H^+	Hydrogen ion
HIV	Human immunodeficiency virus
Hz	Hertz
i.v.	Intravenous
INR	International normalised ratio
IVRA	Intravenous regional anaesthesia
K^+	Potassium ion
Kg (kg)	Kilogram
L	Lumbar (nerve root or dermatome)
l-	Levo (left optical isomer)
LA	Local anaesthetic
LCNT	Lateral cutaneous nerve of the thigh
lido	lidocaine
LMWH	Low molecular weight heparin
mA	Milliampere
mcg	Microgramme
mg	Milligramme
min	Minute
ml	Millilitre
mm	Millimetre
MRI	Magnetic resonance imaging
ms	Millisecond
mV	Millivolt
Na^+	Sodium ion
N/A	Not available
NSAID	Non-steroidal anti-inflammatory drug
PCA	Patient-controlled analgesia
PDPH	Post-dural puncture headache
PNS	Peripheral nerve stimulator
PT	Prothrombin time
PTT	Partial thromboplastin time
prilo	prilocaine
ropiv	ropivacaine
S	Sacral (nerve root or dermatome)
s	Sinister isomer
T	Thoracic (nerve root or dermatome)
$t_{1/2}$	Half-life
UFH	Unfractionated heparin
V	Volt
V_d	Volume of distribution

Further reading

Section 1 Principles and practice

Benefits of regional anaesthesia

1. Liu S, Carpenter RL, Neal JM. Epidural anesthesia and analgesia; their role in postoperative outcome. *Anesthesiology* 1995; 82: 1474–1506
2. Kehlet H. Modification of responses to surgery by neural blockade. In: Cousins MJ, Bridenbaugh PO (eds). *Neural Blockade in Clinical Anaesthesia and Management of Pain, 3rd edition*. Lippincott–Raven, Philadelphia; 1998. 129–175
3. Meissner A, Rolf N, van Aken H. Thoracic epidural anesthesia and the patient with heart disease: benefits, risks and controversies. *Anesth Analg* 1997; 85: 517–528
4. Beattie WS, Badner NH, Choi P. Epidural analgesia reduces postoperative myocardial infarction: a meta-analysis. *Anesth Analg* 2001; 93: 853–858
5. Rodgers A, Walker N et al. Reduction of postoperative mortality and morbidity with epidural or spinal anaesthesia: results from an overview of randomised trials. *Br Med J* 2000; 321: 1493–1497
6. Fischer HBJ. Peripheral nerve blockade in the treatment of pain. *Pain Rev* 1998; 183–202
7. Singelyn FJ, Deyaert M et al. Effects of intravenous patient-controlled analgesia with morphine, continuous epidural analgesia and continuous three-in-one block on postoperative pain and knee rehabilitation after unilateral total knee arthroplasty. *Anesth Analg* 1998; 87: 88–92
8. Capdevila X, Barthelet Y et al. Effects of perioperative analgesic technique on the surgical outcome and duration of rehabilitation after major knee surgery. *Anesthesiology* 1999; 91: 8–15

How to use regional anaesthesia

1. Clinical Practice Guidelines www.esraeurope.org
2. Royal College of Anaesthetists Patient information Project www.youranaesthetic.org
3. Fischer HBJ. Regional anaesthesia – before or after general anaesthesia? *Anaesthesia* 1998; 53: 727–729
4. Bromage PR. A comparison of the hydrochloride and carbon dioxide salts of lidocaine and prilocaine in epidural analgesia. *Acta Anaesthesiol Scand Suppl* 1965; 16: 55–69 (the original description of the Bromage Scale)

Regional anaesthesia equipment

1. BS 5081 Part 2. *Sterile Hypodermic Needles for Single Use*. BSI standards, Milton Keynes; 1987
2. Selander D, Dhuner KG, Lundborg G. Peripheral nerve injury due to injection needles used for regional anaesthesia. *Acta Anaesth Scand* 1977; 21: 182–188
3. Rice AS, McMahon SB. Peripheral nerve injury caused by injection needles used in regional anaesthesia: influence of bevel configuration studied in a rat model. *Br J Anaesth* 1992; 69(5): 433–438
4. Moore DC, Mulroy AF, Thompson GE. Peripheral nerve damage and regional anaesthesia. *Br J Anaesth* 1994; 73(4): 435–436
5. Pither CE, Raj PP, Ford DJ. The use of peripheral nerve stimulators for regional anaesthesia. A review of experimental characteristics, technique, and clinical applications. *Reg Anesth* 1985; 10: 49–58
6. Winnie AP. An 'immobile needle' for nerve blocks. *Anesthesiology* 1969; 31: 577–578
7. Peripheral nerve stimulators for nerve blocks. What are they and how do they work? www.Nysora.com
8. Hadzic A et al. Nerve stimulators used for peripheral nerve blocks vary in their electrical characteristics. *Anesthesiology* 2003; 98: 969–974

Complications of regional anaesthesia

1. Finucane B (ed.). *Complications of Regional Anesthesia*. Churchill Livingstone, New York; 1999
2. Kroll DA, Caplan RA et al. Nerve injury associated with anesthesia. *Anesthesiology* 1990; 72: 202–207

3. Cheney FW et al. Nerve injury associated with anesthesia. *Anesthesiology* 1999; 90: 1062–1069
4. Auroy Y et al. Serious complications related to regional anesthesia. *Anesthesiology* 1997; 87: 479–486
5. Giaufre E et al. Epidemiology and morbidity of regional anesthesia in children. *Anesth Analg* 1996; 83: 904–912
6. Reynolds F. Damage to the conus medullaris following spinal anaesthesia. *Anaesthesia* 2001; 56: 235–247
7. Fettes PD, Wildsmith JAW. Somebody else's nervous system. *Br J Anaesth* 2002; 88: 760–763
8. Borgeat A, Ekatodramis G et al. Acute and non-acute complications associated with interscalene block and shoulder surgery: a prospective study. *Anesthesiology* 2001; 95: 875–880
9. Benumof JL. Permanent loss of cervical spinal cord function associated with interscalene block performed under general anesthesia. *Anesthesiology* 2000; 93: 1541–1544

Pharmacology of local anaesthetic drugs

1. Dollery C (ed.). *Therapeutic drugs, 2nd edition.* Churchill Livingstone, Edinburgh; 1999
2. British National Formulary (September 2003 edition)
3. Rashiq S, Finucane B. Nerve conduction and local anesthetic action. Part 1, Chapter 14. In: *Wylie and Churchill Davidson's Practice of Anesthesia.* Arnold, London; 2003
4. Groban L et al. Cardiac resuscitation after incremental overdosage with lidocaine. Bupivacaine, levobupivacaine and ropivacaine in anesthetised dogs. *Anesth Analg* 2001; 92: 37–43
5. Graf BM et al. Differences in cardiotoxicity of bupivacaine and ropivacaine are the result of physicochemical and stereoselective properties. *Anesth Analg* 2002; 96: 1427–1434

Section 2 Peripheral nerve blocks

Anatomical references

1. Anderson JE. *Grant's Atlas of Anatomy, 7th edition.* The Williams and Wilkins Company, Baltimore; 1978

2. Last RJ. *Anatomy Regional and Applied, 10th edition.* In: Sinnatamby C (ed.). Churchill Livingstone, Edinburgh; 2001
3. Williams PL, Warwick R, Dyson M, Bannister LH (eds). *Gray's Anatomy, 38th edition.* Churchill Livingstone, Edinburgh; 1995

Regional anaesthesia reference texts

1. Scott DB. *Techniques of Regional Anaesthesia, 2nd edition.* Appleton & Lange, Norwalk; 1995
2. Pinnock CA, Fischer HBJ, Jones RP. *Peripheral Nerve Blockade.* Churchill Livingstone, Edinburgh; 1996
3. Cousins MJ, Bridenbaugh PO (eds). *Neural Blockade in Clinical Anesthesia and Management of Pain, 3rd edition.* Lippincott, Philadelphia; 1998
4. Brown DL. *Atlas of Regional Anesthesia, 2nd edition.* WB Saunders Company, Philadelphia; 1999
5. Wildsmith JA, Armitage EN, McClure JH (eds). *Principles and Practice of Regional Anaesthesia, 3rd edition.* Churchill Livingstone, Edinburgh; 2003

The lower extremity

Femoral nerve

1. Winnie AP, Rammamurthy S, Durrani A. The inguinal paravascular technic of lumbar plexus anaesthesia; the '3 in 1' block. *Anesth Analg* 1973; 52: 989–996
2. Marhofer P, Nasel C et al. Magnetic resonance imaging of the distribution of local anaesthetic during the three-in-one block. *Anesth Analg* 2000; 90: 119–124

Sciatic nerve

1. Labat G. *Regional Anesthesia; Its Technic and Clinical Application.* WB Saunders, Philadelphia and London; 1922. 291–299
2. Raj PP et al. New single position supine approach to sciatic–femoral nerve block. *Anesth Analg* 1975; 54: 489
3. Guardini R et al. Sciatic nerve block: a new lateral approach. *Acta Anaesthesiol Scand* 1985; 29: 515
4. Vloka JD et al. Anatomic considerations for sciatic nerve block in the popliteal fossa through the lateral approach. *Reg Anesth* 1996; 21: 414–418

5. Hadzic A, Vloka JD. Comparison of posterior versus lateral approaches to the block of the sciatic nerve in the popliteal fossa. *Anesthesiology* 1998; 88: 1480–1486
6. Wassef MR. Sustentaculum tali approach to the tibial nerve. *Anaesthesia* 1991; 46: 841–842

Lumbar plexus

1. Chayen D, Nathan H, Chayen M. The psoas compartment block. *Anesthesiology* 1976; 45: 95–99
2. Farny J, Drolet P, Girard M. Anatomy of the posterior approach to the lumbar plexus block. *Can Anaesth* 1994; 41: 480–485
3. Capdevila X et al. Continuous psoas compartment block for postoperative analgesia after total hip arthroplasty: new landmarks, technical guidelines and clinical evaluation. *Anesth Analg* 2002; 94: 1606–1613
4. De Biasi P et al. Continuous lumbar plexus block: use of radiography to determine catheter tip location. *RAPM* 2003; 28: 135–139

The abdomen and thorax

1. Richardson J, Lonnqvist PA. Thoracic paravertebral block. *Br J Anaesth* 1998; 81: 230–238
2. Richardson J et al. A prospective randomised comparison of preoperative and balanced epidural or paravertebral bupivacaine on post-thoracotomy pain, pulmonary function and stress responses. *Br J Anaesth* 1999; 83: 387–392

The upper extremity

1. Winnie AP. Plexus anaesthesia. *Perivascular Techniques of Brachial Plexus Block*. Schultz, Copenhagen; Vol 1, 1983
2. Winnie AP, Collins VJ. The subclavian perivascular technique of brachial plexus anaesthesia. *Anesthesiology* 1964; 25: 353–363
3. De Andres J et al. Peripheral nerve stimulation in the practice of brachial plexus anesthesia: a review. *Reg Anesth Pain Med* 2001; 26: 478–483
4. Neal JM et al. Brachial plexus anesthesia: essentials of our current understanding. *Reg Anesth Pain Med* 2002; 27: 402–428

5. Mehrkens HH, Geiger PK. Continuous brachial plexus blockade via the vertical infraclavicular approach. *Anaesthesia* 1998; 53: 19S–20S
6. Wasseff MR. Suprascapular nerve block. A new approach for the management of frozen shoulder. *Anaesthesia* 1992; 47: 120–123

Ophthalmic surgery

1. Smith GB, Hamilton RC, Carr CA. *Ophthalmic Anaesthesia – A Practical Handbook.* Arnold, London; 1996
2. Joint College Guidelines, Local Anaesthesia for Intraorbital Surgery. The Royal College of Anaesthetists and The Royal College of Ophthalmologists 2001
3. Kumar CM, Dodds C, Fanning GL. *Ophthalmic Anaesthesia.* Swets and Zeitlinger b.v. Lisse; 2002

The head, neck and airway

1. Stoneham MD, Knighton JD. Regional anaesthesia for carotid endarterectomy. *Br J Anaesth* 1999; 82: 910–919
2. Tanganakul C et al. Local versus general for carotid endarterectomy 2000. *Cochrane Database Syst Rev*
3. Davies MJ et al. Superficial and deep cervical plexus blocks for carotid artery surgery: a prospective study of 1000 blocks. *Reg Anesth* 1997; 22: 442–446

Continuous peripheral nerve catheter techniques

1. Rosenblatt R. Continuous femoral anesthesia for lower extremity surgery. *Anesth Analg* 1980; 59: 631–632
2. Smith B, Fischer HBJ, Scott PV. Continuous sciatic nerve block. *Anaesthesia* 1984; 39: 155–157
3. Fischer HBJ, Peters TM et al. Peripheral nerve catheterisation in the management of terminal cancer pain. *Reg Anesth* 1996; 21: 482–485
4. Singelyn F, Aye F, Gouverneur JM. Continuous popliteal sciatic nerve block: an original technique to provide postoperative analgesia after foot surgery. *Anesth Analg* 1997; 84: 383–386
5. Borgeat A, Schappi B et al. Patient-controlled analgesia after major shoulder surgery. *Anesthesiology* 1997; 87: 1343–1347

Section 3 Central neuraxial blocks

Applied anatomy of the central neuraxis

1. Agur A, Dalley A. *Grant's Atlas of Anatomy, 10th edition.* Lippincott Williams and Wilkins, Baltimore; 2004
2. Last RJ. *Anatomy Regional and Applied, 10th edition.* In: Sinnatamby C (ed.). Churchill Livingstone, Edinburgh; 2001
3. Williams PL (ed.). *Gray's Anatomy, 39th edition.* Elsevier, London; 2004

Applied physiology of the spinal cord

1. Brown DL. *Atlas of Regional Anesthesia, 2nd edition.* WB Saunders Company, Philadelphia; 1999
2. Wildsmith JA, Armitage EN, McClure JH (eds). *Principles and Practice of Regional Anaesthesia, 3rd edition.* Churchill Livingstone, Edinburgh; 2003

Indications for central neuraxial blockade

Spinal

1. Greene NM, Brull SJ. *Physiology of Spinal Anesthesia, 4th edition.* Williams and Wilkins, Baltimore; 1993
2. Stienstra R, Veering B. Intrathecal drug spread: is it controllable? *Reg Anesth Pain Med* 1998; 23: 347–351
3. Bannister J, McCLure JH, Wildsmith JAW. Effect of glucose concentration on the intrathecal spread of 0.5% bupivacaine. *Br J Anaesth* 1990; 64: 232–234
4. Denny NM, Selander DE. Continuous spinal anaesthesia. *Br J Anaesth* 1998; 81: 590–597
5. Caplan RA et al. Unexpected cardiac arrest during spinal anesthesia. A closed claims analysis of predisposing factors. *Anesthesiology* 1988; 68: 5–11
6. Pollard JB. Cardiac arrest during spinal anaesthesia: common mechanisms and strategies for prevention. *Anesth Analg* 2001; 92: 252–256

Epidural

1. Covino BG, Scott DB, McClure JH. *Handbook of Epidural Anaesthesia and Analgesia.* Mediglobe Fribourg; 1999
2. Cousins MJ, Veering BT. Epidural neural blockade. In: Cousins MJ, Bridenbaugh PO (eds). *Neural Blockade in Clinical Anesthesia and Management of Pain, 3rd edition.* Lippincott, Philadelphia; 1998. 243–323

Caudal

1. Armitage EN. Caudal block in children. *Anaesthesia* 1979; 34: 396

Index

Note: page numbers in italic refer to illustrations and tables; *n.b.* is nerve block